CARNIVORE DIET

Enjoy succulent meat recipes, to strengthen the body, increase muscle mass and lose weight

Mark Greger

CONTENTS

INTRODUCTION

This is the right book for you if you're someone who loves a juicy steak, or just about any type of meat. Here, we will delve deeply into a diet that challenges what you know about nutrition and health and allows you to explore new possibilities. The diet is the Carnivore Diet, as the title suggests. A lot of you may or not be conversant with what this diet is all about, but nevertheless it will all be explained in this book.

The Carnivore Diet's main emphasis is on consuming only meat from any source and not eating plant foods. This diet has recently gained considerable popularity, and the strong motivation behind this diet is usually weight loss. Most people follow this diet to resolve some form of autoimmune system issue, where diets consisting of meat are beneficial.

Since attempting the Paleo and the Ketogenic diet, a lot of people have been trying the Carnivore Diet. The Paleo Diet is, as you might know, a caveman diet that focuses on eating fresh foods like our ancestors ate during the caveman era. It eliminates all processed foods, grains, milk products, sugars, etc. that were not available at that time.

On the other hand, the Ketogenic Diet focuses on a significant reduction in carbohydrates from the diet with a high fat intake and a moderate protein intake. The diet is suitable for people who want a higher intake of protein and wish to limit their intake of fats or carbs.

Once you read the book, you'll understand exactly what the Carnivore Diet entails. The meat only diet is pretty much self-explanatory, but you can work with a few gray areas to create a proper healthy diet for yourself. A lot of people have tried this diet and if properly followed, you will benefit from losing weight and getting healthier.

If you're a lover of meat, the diet is like a dream come true for you. It is best to approach the diet and nutrition with an open mind, even if that means questioning things about which you are "positive" on a regular basis. The body changes with age, even if you were right.

My aim is to stimulate discussion about a Carnivore Diet and share tips for doing so, as well as tools that you can further explore. I don't have all the answers and I hope you approach this book with an open mind.

I don't say everyone should adhere to a strict meat-only diet, either. I don't think there is enough evidence to back that up yet. It's up to you to plot out what makes you feel best, until much more (and better) studies are done. Maybe you're going to thrive on a strict, meat-only diet or maybe you're wired to work best with just a meat-heavy diet, or not even that. In any case, the following pages will give you some insight as to why I started following a Carnivore Diet, how I did it, tips for change and (of course) recipes to get you started.

What is the Diet of a Carnivore?

Often known as a zero-carb diet, a carnivorous diet or the all-meat diet, the Carnivorous Diet has one simple working principle; you can only eat meat! Essentially, as long as you follow the diet, you are supposed to eat almost nothing but meat for every single meal every day. This diet won't dictate your servings, calories, diet timings or macro percentages. You are allowed to eat anytime you are hungry, and to feel full as much as you need to.

It's exactly what you'd think about eating a Carnivore Diet: you eat animal products (and by-products).

You don't eat plants (fruits, vegetables, nuts, seeds, grains, or legumes).

The Carnivore Diet is also commonly termed as a "zero-carb" diet, or "all-meat" diet, although zero carb is a bit misleading since olive oil is a zero-carb plant, and therefore not on a Diet. Eggs also carry a trace of carbohydrates. There are also trace amounts of starch in full-fat foods, such as cheese and whipping cream. So, if you are consuming a so-called "zero-carb" diet, it may have trace amounts of carbohydrates depending on the foods you eat.

Nonetheless, some people on a carnivorous diet find such methods to be hair splitting and they call it a zero-carb diet because it basically has no carbohydrates.

There are some gray areas that a diet follower can tailor to match his choices.

Many individuals, for example, add foods such as cream or cheese to their diet while others impose a maximum ban on eating anything other than meat. You can consume animal-sourced food, which includes meat, eggs or dairy, according to diet guidelines. Such foods can contain as much protein and fat as you need, but carbohydrates should be omitted from the diet.

Thanks to the carbohydrate-eliminating factor the Carnivore Diet is especially beneficial. There are some places around the world where people only live on zero carbohydrates and eat according to the Carnivore Diet instead. It's not because they're following a fad diet, but as far back as they can remember, it's a practice they've followed. When you think of living only on meat, fish, etc. with absolutely no grains or such carbohydrates, it might sound extreme to you. This is mostly because your usual diet contains grains as a staple and you've been told they're healthy for your heart. Evidence, however, indicates that the advent of refined carbohydrates is what caused a huge increase in people's rates of diabetes, obesity, tooth cavities and atherosclerosis. That's why a lot of people try to cut carbohydrates from their diet these days.

Another major factor is the excessive consumption of carbon is a major cause of weight gain. To be honest, removing carbs will work for some people whilst it may not work for some. You should customize your diet to suit the needs of your body. Reducing carbohydrates in your diet can help you with weight loss and other health problems, but it's a macro that needs to be regulated and doesn't always need to be eliminated completely.

Many studies have been carried out to see the effects of a low carbohydrate diet on humans. Which show that that carbs improves mental performance, increases physical endurance, helps digestion and also decreases body inflammation. A low carb diet is good for cardiovascular health, too.

Another benefit is that it increases vitality while raising the cravings for unhealthy food. Together, all these factors show that a no-carb Carnivore Diet can improve health, and also reduce your weight. This diet is just one of the strict variations of low-carb or high-fat diets like diets like Paleo and Keto. In this carnivore version, there is a complete elimination of this macro from the diet instead of merely reducing the carbs.

As we mentioned earlier, the Carnivore Diet has cultural precedence. For example, in Eskimo groups, their diet consisted mostly of fish, walrus, or whales as a diet made from high-fat animals. Even in Africa's Masai region the diet is predominantly meat with milk. Such people have also shown relatively low levels of bad cholesterol and low rates of cardiovascular diseases.

If you want real researched proof of the Carnivore Diet's effects, there are unfortunately not enough long-term formal studies yet completed; however, there are many trending forums online that you can go check to find out more about the real-life effects of this diet.

Many of the people who followed the Carnivore Diet leave testimonials or feedback on how they've turned out. You can always use these to judge whether or not the diet suits your needs; however, in the end, the best way to know for certain is to follow and experience the diet yourself. If you're not a fan of salad greens but enjoy your meats, this diet can be pretty tempting.

How would I eat on a Carnivore Diet?

There are several ways to approach the Carnivore Diet.

You'd say, "How's that? It sounds pretty simple...... eat animals, and don't eat plants. Got it. "Yes, that is the most basic form of diet. But you do have a lot of options from there.

A Carnivore Diet/meal plan can include any of the following meals: Beef, Chicken, Buffalo, Eggs, Turkey, Duck, Pork, Fish, Mutton / Lamb, Rabbit, Venison / Elk, Goat, Oyster, Lobster, Crab, Shrimp, Squid, Octopus, Offal (liver, kidney, tongue, heart, etc.), Snake, Alligator, Frog legs, and Dairy (wholly fat options are best: cheese, yogurt, milk, heavy cream, butter, and ghee). That's a lot of choices. In fact, there are various ways of preparing these foods for a variety of meat-heavy versatility. Roasted, stewed, fried, steamed, seared, etc. Two things worth noting: gravitating to a beef-heavy diet is popular among Carnivore Dieters over time. It did happen to me, too. It's simple, delicious and the desire for variety is just beginning to diminish. I have read about Carnivore Dietitians who only eat beef and drink water. This is it. There are others who eat only ribeye steaks and drink water to be even more specific.

Most carnivorous dieters avoid dairy, or only rarely eat it. It's always full-fat (cheese, butter, ghee, or heavy cream), if they do have milk products.

BEEF AND DAIRY

Because it's nutrient dense and extremely satisfying, many Carnivore Dieters eat mostly beef, especially fatty cuts, over other animal products. High nutrition and satiety are absolutely key to the fatty part, so I never trim the fat and I eat it all.

Like the other carnivorous dieters, after a while I too migrated to prefer mostly beef. I needed variety at first. I was afraid of getting bored so I was eating pork, chicken, fish and milk products.

However, over the course of two months eating carnivore, I noticed I mostly desired beef, particularly fatty rib-eye steaks. God, how I loved those fats. I ate less pork, more dairy products and more chicken over time. They always made appearances, as did offal (when my attitude is good enough for nutrition), but they were not the rule for me.

As for dairy, allergies are the main reasons many carnivores go without it, or just plain not feeling as optimal with added dairy. They may get cheese on a beef patty on occasion, but they go without dairy for most days. There are times when I come home and I haven't eaten in seven hours. I'm hungry, and I still have dinner to cook. For me the perfect snack is an ounce of cheese, or two. This takes away the feeling of hunger entirely before I cook up a proper pound of ground beef or steak.

Dairy was a clever choice for me as I transitioned to the Carnivore Diet. It's delicious, and satisfying.

DO YOU NEED VEGGIES?

Research on this is surprisingly lacking. It's absolutely possible we don't. Most experts say carbohydrates are not necessary, while no one says protein and fats are not important. One can obtain vitamins and minerals from animal sources. That leaves the question of particular phytonutrients (plant compounds), and science has just started asking the somewhat heretical question of whether these are essential in a plant-free diet.

What we do know is that, throughout the world, there are people and certain civilizations throughout history who mainly subsisted on a diet that was very low in carbs. And there were periods in many cultures when carbohydrates were only available during certain times of the year. So, it looks like there were people who survived without eating carbohydrates every day for generations.

CARNIVORE DIET SOUNDS WEIRD. IS IT DANGEROUS?

I know what those people wonder about. Is it weird? Is that threatening?

It was new to me, at first. Eating just meat runs counter to traditional dietary wisdom, that says, "you need to eat a lot of vegetables, fiber, and grains.

The Inuit, Plains Indians, Mongolians, and Masai are just a few of the more well-known meat-heavy groups of people (meaning they most often consume a diet of "only meat"). The bison has been famously called the "staff of life" for the North American Plains Indians since prehistoric times, and they lived primarily on this and other game animals.

These cultures thrived too. This means we have meat-eating civilizations and their good health information and accounts. They had a lack of most of the diseases we are suffering from in today's world where people eat a lot of plants, particularly grains. Which made me irritated. What if people don't even need to eat plants?

There's more to wellness though than just food. These people, hunched over a computer, didn't eat meat off the bone all day. They were very healthy-many of them were nomadic tribes pursuing the herds of game-which means they got a lot of exercise. Their lives were dependent on a lot of walking or running. Diet is important in terms of health and longevity, but not the only factor. It is one of many things that I have in my toolkit.

Context is important when we are thinking about "plants." Note, this is about the entire kingdom of plants, not just fruits and vegetables. If somebody eats an omnivore diet of meat and grains, then replacing the grains with fruits and vegetables will offer absolutely better nutrition. But the question of whether we can get everything we need from meat–that is, whether we actually need any plants (grains, fruits, vegetables, etc.) instead of eating a completely Carnivore Diet... well... it defies conventional wisdom, but at the moment I'm not convinced we need plants anymore. I assume that animal products could be used to get everything we need.

Highsteaks.com provides an amusing article which asks if you need veggies to be safe. Here are some of the highlights (although the whole article is worth reading).

Animal food supplies all of the micronutrients a person needs.

Animal products are some of the most nutrient-dense foods. They are our best (and often only) source of vitamin A (retinol), DHA / EPA, and Vitamin B12, together with lesser-known nutrients such as choline, creatine, and carnosine.

In animal foods there are plenty of nutrients we NEED that can only be found in animal foods, but none in plants that are unavailable in animal foods.

Plants have plenty of nutrients, but they aren't a "healthy" source because they come with plenty of "anti-nutrients" that bind to the same receptors and minimize body absorption, or are killed by cooking, or are unavailable without some added fats.

If you want, you can eat veggies-not because they are "good," but because they can be delicious... (And to keep Mom happy.)

Is A Carnivore Diet DANGEROUS?

To my best knowledge, I don't think eating a Carnivore Diet is dangerous, based on much research. Although there is a scarcity of clinical research, I have come to this conclusion based on 1) the anthropological evidence (above), 2) the anecdotal success of other people with the diet, and 3) based on my own experience with it to date.

On the other hand, I consider processed foods and refined sugars as the harmful foods, not meat. Eating lots of steaks doesn't make me scared. I eat this way because when I do, I simply feel better and I seem to be able to stay in good shape and maintain muscle mass with less exercise than when I was on an omnivore diet.

CHAPTER 1: UNDERSTANDING THE ORIGINS OF THE CARNIVORE DIET

There is a simple reason behind its success according to the people who advocate the advantages of the Carnivore Diet. The reason our ancestors tended to eat most of the time because it took a lot of energy to harvest fruits and vegetables. Hunting and eating meat was considerably more energy-efficient. Because of this carnivorous diet followed by our ancestors, our bodies evolved in a way that when our diet is meat-centric they run at the most optimal level. This is one of the main myths underpinning the Carnivore Diet.

There are many examples in recorded history of people from a variety of racial, cultural or even regional backgrounds who survived a meat-centric diet and remained very healthy throughout their years. On the other hand, no society or civilization has been noted for generations of following a purely vegan diet. There must be a reason behind which most people have preferred meat as the main component of their diets throughout the ages.

There's a lot of stigma against meat these days. Most people seem to support a vegetarian or vegan or even a fruit diet free of any meat or animal-derived food. We are taught that meat is the reason for clogging of the arteries, weight gain, high cholesterol levels, constipation, etc. So you should give up meat and adopt a diet based entirely on plants; however, no society has people who have lived healthily from infancy to old age on a vegan diet.

When you look at it anthropologically, the real-world examples of different cultures adopting a particular diet are much more relevant than any scientific studies done to explain something. The fact that humans thrived on the Carnivore Diet throughout the ages is a much more compelling testimony that the knowledge collected through a scientific study was performed over a few weeks on several individuals. The former is a more practical way of looking at the diet than the latter, including a group of people who have been consuming more meat than normal for some time while doing a research.

Studies have been conducted to demonstrate clearly that a diet with less animal products is safer than a diet with more of it; however, these researches have mostly failed to prove this since a non-vegetarian culture is no less safe than a vegetarian society in any way. Animal foods are absolutely essential to a human being's health. If you look at different groups all over the world and also study their history, you will notice that every healthy community survives on at least a few, if not a lot, of animal foods. There is no healthy group of people wholly independent of food from animal sources.

As we mentioned before, in the world two specific groups are being used as a prime example of a healthy carnivorous community. The first group is the

Eskimos, who almost exclusively eat meat and fat. People living in the Arctic regions only saw a change in their diet around the latter part of the 1800s, when extensive trade routes were being built. This provided them with access to sugar, flour, and other European foods that were then introduced into their original diet. However, they were healthier on the diet, which consisted primarily of animal protein with fat, before this change in diet.

The second group is the African Masai people, who eat very little plant food and mostly survive on meat, milk, and even animal blood. The herdsmen from these African regions consume more meat when they are between 14 and 30 years old since these are their warrior years. Additional meat was deemed essential to strengthening muscles, and would therefore be helpful to a warrior. Nevertheless, it should be noted that the old cultures which adopted this form of meat-centered diet did so in order to adapt to certain severe environmental factors. Most of the groups worldwide that followed a carnivorous diet live in desert, arctic or sub-arctic areas. In such areas the food is scarce and food availability is also unpredictable.

Many other communities also survive on a meat-based diet; for example-the Canadian Arctic region's Inuit. Their diet mainly consists of salmon, walrus, whale, and seal meat. The people of Chukotka in the Russian Arctic live on a diet of sea creatures, caribou meat, and fish. The Samburu and the Rendille people in East Africa have survived on a meat and milk diet for years. In Mongolia the nomads of the Steppe usually eat dairy products and meat every day. The Sioux are considered to have had buffalo meat as the staple of their diet in southern Dakota. For the Brazilian Gauchos, beef is the major part of their meals.

As you will notice, a Carnivore Diet has been used all over the world for a very long time and despite the stigma against meat these people have enjoyed healthy lives for generations. The myth that remains in the American diet about saturated fat and meat cholesterol is completely discredited. The groups of people who eat meat filled diet in the Arctic and African tribes have no recorded past instances of heart disease or such ailments and these only increased when modern foods were introduced into their diets.

When you take time to look at the diet of the Arctic region's ethnic groups, you'll see that they're hardly eating any amount of fruit or vegetables throughout the year. Doesn't that make you wonder how they manage to survive or live healthy lives? You probably doubt that they then received sufficient amounts of essential vitamins and minerals in their diet; however, as they do today, they have lived like this for a very long time and have thrived on this diet.

One of the famous studies supporting the Carnivore Diet is one conducted by a Cleveland dentist named Weston A. Price. He started a research that he carried out for nearly a decade on the subject. He has learned from his experience how most people suffered from dental problems and other metabolic conditions. He noticed all of the health problems and even the facial deformities that continued to increase in the number of patients he had seen.

He was curious about the origin of these problems because he believed that God was not the one who would allow his people to suffer this sort of suffering. This curiosity and interest led him to investigate the root cause of all these illnesses. There was no one else at that point 60 years ago who had given this considerable thought. He was the only one who aimed to study different civilizations around the world and learn from different people about the cause of the health problems he came across.

He went to Africa, Australia and many more places around the world from the Swiss Region. He was surprised by this and was very curious about how without any help from modern medicine, they could be in such good health. The key to all of his questions lies in those isolated ethnic groups' eating habits. His findings were that they all had a diet that barely contained any plant products and it was mostly based on products of animal origin. His study was just another proof that meat is, and should not be eliminated, a very healthy component of human diet. A meat-centered diet contains adequate amounts of the nutrients and minerals required for optimal physical health.

Another research to remember is one that was done in Point Hope, Alaska, about 40 years ago. The place is very isolated, so they were still on a very meat-focused diet for this reason. The study was published in 1972 and gave different observations based on their diet and their health. It said Point Hope's people were one of the very few surviving groups on the Eskimo diet that had survived. Their average daily calorie intake was 3,000 kcal per person, and half of that was fat, while about 35 per cent was protein. Only a maximum of 20 per cent of their calories were derived from carbohydrates in the form of starch from animals.

Their diet had scarcely any grains, and when a little is added to tea or coffee, that was the only time saccharose is ingested. Evidence has shown that Point Hope residents have an approximately 10-fold lower rate of heart diseases compared to the rest of the general population in the US. From this you can see that eating doesn't have a negative impact on your cardiovascular health as is said these days. Yet between the years 1906 and 1919, Vilhjalmur Stefansson conducted another meat based dietary research on the Inuit people and found they were even stronger and healthier than he had imagined.

CHAPTER 2: THE TECHNICAL ASPECTS OF THE ABOUT CARNIVORE DIET

Probably, our ancestors did not think much about nutrition. They acted on instinct, living in the sun naturally, eating wild foods and sleeping beneath the stars. But there are signs that they knew that eating these foods was advantageous even if they did not know the difference between Omega-3 and Omega-6 fats, or why the animal source of Vitamin A (retinol) is more bioavailable and beneficial to humans than the plant form (beta-carotene).

They praised organ meats such as liver and kidneys, and knew about eating bone marrow— whether instinctively or through generations of passed-on wisdom. Sure, they certainly spent most of their time trying to obtain calories and they definitely didn't understand the science behind the fact that wild animals store the essential vitamins we need in their liver, fat stores and marrow. But nature and acquired knowledge had a way of compelling them to consume the nutrients they needed most.

"Hunting man is a connoisseur of fats and has a definite sequence of tastes in the various fats according to their origin in different parts of the body," Adventurer Vilhjalmur Stefansson wrote in his seminal 1956 book *The Fat of the Land* about the Inuit preferences for caribou.

"The marrows are best, and range in excellence from the hip and shoulder joints down — the farther down, the better... The descending ratings are: the fat from behind the eye, the kidney fat, the fat from the brisket near the bone, the fat from the ribs and other parts where it is mixed with the lean. Last comes the back fat.

"These people may not have known that vitamin A is important for the eye health when searching for fat and organs. But many have come to understand that eyeballs — a food high in vitamin A — would fix eye problems. We also understood what foods to eat at various developmental stages, which we know has been done by different groups. They will feed these things to nursing mothers, couples trying to conceive, individuals living with the illness, and elderly community members.

When it comes to medicine and hydration, we see similar practices— even among communities that still live apart from modern society today.

Indigenous groups living deep within the Amazon can't tell you about biochemistry and other processes that regulate the response of the immune system.

But they know exactly what kind of tree bark can help treat hernia and what vines they can cut to acquire a safe drinking water source.

In this sense, their perception of the natural world around them, and especially their diet, was a bit mechanistic. Collective wisdom has been learnt and passed down over thousands of years and hundreds of generations.

This practical knowledge became essential for their survival and health. It's a shame it got lost in just a couple of decades.

That was their "conventional wisdom," but it was somehow mostly lost in time, replaced by decades of rapid change that gave some invaluable scientific insight — especially on bacteria and pathogens— but also largely distorted by an underlying drive to feed as many people as possible, as cheaply as possible.

Yet optimal human health fell by the wayside for the adult. From the top it all went towards the goal of preventing acute nutrient deficiencies among a population of 330 million people. And all the advice is embroidered in the underlying biased view that mass food production and transportation are necessary. FDA recommendations only consider that preservatives and additives are actually toxic, rather than beginning from the point of view that none of this should be present in our food!

Massive corporations have come to dominate supplying food. Their objective was not to raise animals which provide the best nutrition for people. They wanted to raise animals the cheapest way they could. This meant keeping cows indoors on relatively small feedlots, and pushing them to eat the cheapest available feed.

We were given corn and soy drenched with agrochemicals that would help these crops grow more quickly. They then pumped steroids and hormones into the cows to get even more meat per cow. And they had to pump them full of antibiotics to keep the animals from contracting diseases and dying before slaughter due to this horrible lifestyle.

The same was true for plant foods. The emphasis has always been on optimizing yields and engineering crops resistant to drought and blight.

Good intentions— helping communities escape past famines that killed so many people. This was awesome! But corporate profit targets would overtake those noble goals, and plant nutrient content would plummet over the decades.

Why? For what? The response to that is always money.

Mark Schatzker in his book the Dorito Effect, discusses how dramatically the scientists who conducted the research dubbed "The Dilution Effect" has taken away from plant foods through modern farming methods and crop engineering. The following are just a few of the many improvements illustrated. "The kale of the 1950s had twice as much riboflavin (Vitamin B2) as modern kale. Cauliflower in the 1950s had double the thiamine (Vitamin B1). And asparagus in the 1950s had nearly three times as much as ascorbic acid (Vitamin C)... It was as if modern products had been nutritionally dumbed down. "Also, the role of government in all of this is not motivated by improving people's health. We basically evaluate all the unhealthy parts of the process and determine whether this chemical, that hormone, or some other antibiotic can cause the user serious harm.

They're not saying the obvious: None of that should be in our food! And they don't warn people that the end product is beef, beyond all the harmful ingredients, which is much lower in the nutrients that we need to live in optimum health.

The deterioration in food quality is the biggest factor in our health decline, as we will address much more in chapters to come. For now, the key message from this brief history to remember is this: We've discarded everything we've learned over the past hundred thousand years. And while it might have helped provide more productive sustenance for billions of people, it is now undermining our individual health.

There's no longer a need to worry about caloric scarcity in much of the United States, at least among almost everybody reading this book. The opposite is the problem. Overconsumption is the rule now as we have too much access to unnaturally appetizing food.

But even though people are eating more and more, they are getting less and less of what they actually need. Previous humans sometimes went days— sometimes weeks— without food. Without a snack, we cannot go on for three hours.

No one believes sweets and potato chips have any nutritional value, but people do believe that brown rice, fruits, and grocery-store yogurt give them all they need. People even think in very simple terms— saying "this is safe" as they eat a sugar-filled smoothie, but it has no nutrients to speak about — and then go about their day without knowing that many of the main building blocks of actual health are lacking.

What does it miss? It can be a lot depending on what they eat.

But there are a couple of absolutely vital components that people need.

These are the different vitamins, and one fatty acid, that you really need to prioritize and appreciate if you are to maintain your optimum health. There are more things without doubt that you have to get to achieve this target. But by prioritizing these three vitamin types, and one fatty acid, the rest will mostly come naturally into place.

This is our scientific response; we know that these nutrients are essential to health. The logical response is related to ancestral diets, these animal nutrients have been present throughout all indigenous groups.

To make feeding simpler and take some of the mystery out of it, this book begins with these, "The Fundamental Four," which will form the basis of nutrient density. This doesn't necessarily mean the others are less significant. But these four are often poorly understood and lacking.

If you start here, get back to the basics, and start getting each of these basic nutrients, you'll be on your way to eating — and feeling — better quickly.

Before delving into the specific vitamins and fat we need, understanding the core philosophy behind that diet is important. The goal of the Carnivore Diet is to eat the most nutritionally dense foods (from animals) possible while avoiding anything that can be harmful (by causing inflammation, introducing anti-nutrients, harming our intestines or disrupting the natural mechanisms in our bodies in general).

It means eating high-quality animal foods, and the good news is that we can get all the nutrients we need without a lot of calories being eaten. Through eating the right things (like liver, some fish and the right cheese) we will have gotten all we need.

Yet, of course, beyond nutrients, we also need enough calories to fuel our bodies to stay alive and enough protein to regenerate cells, tissues, and muscles. Those two areas become the focus after we meet our dietary targets.

The key goal will be to reduce inflammation while eating. In a later chapter, we will cover that deeper— but this is one of the key reasons why plant foods are not just unnecessary, but potentially harmful. We'll also dig deeper into why I don't eat plant foods later in the book.

But we need to understand why before we really explain what we should eat.

Why do so many different nutrients matter? When planning your diet, what nutrients should you be concentrating on? What are the growing shortcomings, and how do you avoid missing out on the things your body needs most?

We're about to start exploring all that right now. Yet, at the same time, it's not a lecture on genetics. My aim in the next few pages is to give an overview of the primary vitamins and nutrients I think should be the nutritional foundation of your diet and the main reasons you need to get them. I want to give you the concrete information to help you understand why you need these nutrients. With so much scientific knowledge and so many research studies, I don't want to dwell on that, so that tomorrow you forget it all.

This is why I will concentrate on the processes within the body and continue to express how important it was for our indigenous ancestors to eat such nutrients. Hopefully, by taking this approach, you will come to understand why I placed such a target in my diet for getting these specific nutrients.

Vitamin A - If you look at a standard nutrition guide online, it will inform you that vitamin A is important to keep your teeth, bones, soft tissue, mucous membranes and skin healthy. It will mention the importance of vitamin A in eye health and inform you that its scientific (chemical) names (retinol, retinal, and retinoic acid) are related to its function in producing pigments in the eye's retina. You may learn that a deficiency in vitamin A can result in blindness.

While these factors are of course important, much more needs to be known.

Along with many other fat-soluble vitamins we will be addressing, vitamin A is vital to cell differentiation and gene expression— the mechanism through which each cell in the body is essentially made.

Because this cycle is the foundation of all life, the value of these vitamins in human biology is understated. Many people are going to go their entire lives without even knowing what this is or how our diet can affect those functions.

Cell expression switches genes on and off in the simplest terms to control what cells the body needs, and cell differentiation is the operation of those cells being specialized cells (such as white blood cells or stem cells). Genes are what define all the functional control characteristics of our bodies.

The fact that most diets lack the nutrients key for such a basic cell function can probably explain most people's poor health. All these fat-soluble vitamins are connected together in complex biochemical chains that include other vitamins, minerals, nutrients, fatty acids, and almost anything that enters your body.

So while the impact of vitamin A on this cycle is not special, it has a major role to play. Retinoic acid in the sense of gene expression actively controls hundreds of genes in the body, including differentiation of stem cells (meaning the output of stem cells), and differentiation of germ cells in embryonic development. Ultimately it has a role to play in controlling over 500 genes!

And most people don't eat almost enough vitamin A to ensure all these essential processes are properly regulated. Yet they believe they are because of a completely different type of poor regulation: from the U.S. government this time.

The developed Recommended Dietary Allowances (RDA) and Dietary Reference Intakes (DRI) allow for the labeling of beta-carotene from plant foods as vitamin A (in the form of retinol activity equivalents, or RAE) through the Institute of Medicine (IOM). But this material, also known as "Provitamin A," is not what our body actually requires. Such carotenoids need to be transformed by the body into the functional retinal type (or "preformed vitamin A"), and the conversion rates will vary significantly from person to person. In addition, many people only transform beta-carotene in very small amounts.

And this mechanism can be further disrupted in a number of ways, including certain gene variations between humans and compounds in plant foods, which hinder certain enzymes active in conversions.

In short, (1) the animal portion of vitamin A is the most bioavailable for our body and (2) some of us can only obtain it in high quantities from a few specific sources (i.e., liver and high quality egg yolks). You may be very wrong if you eat carrots and kale on a daily basis and believe all those carotenoids are doing the job.

All this also spurs another key point to remember about the RDAs: They have been created to help avoid deficiencies in 97.5 percent of the total population— not to encourage optimal health. In fact, they have only been revised once (in 2016) since its establishment in 1968.

How exactly are we taking advice from a government body that updates its information every 50 years? And should we just try to avoid deficiencies or, indeed, optimize our intake?

Really, it the importance of vitamin A cannot be overestimated. And just as all of the fat-soluble vitamins are important, starting to eat foods high in vitamin A is one way many people can almost immediately create a noticeable difference in their health.

VITAMIN A: SOURCES & PREPARATION -- Out of the so-called "superfoods" declared by "experts" and magazine articles, nothing could be better to eat than liver. Whether it's cow, lamb, chicken, duck, other birds, cod, or other fish, liver is the only natural food source that's really high in Vitamin A.

With that being said, it is alright to say that not every individual in every tribe could get enough liver to eat. A growing animal has only one, and the muscle meat, fat, and even other organs are not that large relative to their bodies. But even small ocean fishes, shellfishes, and insects either have small vitamin A stores in their livers, or they're just much higher in vitamin A than the foods we eat now. So even when the big-game hunting didn't go so well our ancestors could get by.

This was great as people don't even need all that much in general.

Depending on body size, only 100 grams of liver a week are possibly appropriate. That said, they should prioritize consumption early on. Eating more is probably a good idea because the majority of people living on a Standard American Diet will have deficiencies. And this refers not only to vitamin A, but to most of the essential nutrients. Even though indigenous people in the past had adequate levels starting in the womb, you will have to adjust for some lost time in the beginning process.

Cod liver supplements are a choice in our modern days for people who don't like liver, or who find it hard to source locally. And this is not just a new diet fad like most herbal or major retailer's supplements.

All of your grandparents are likely to tell you about the awful taste when they were force-fed spoonfuls of cod liver or fish oil. Luckily, the varieties of today have a better flavour, but for a long, long time people have relied on fish liver oil.

"Scandanavian fishermen also believe in the almost mystical benefit of cod or halibut liver oil and some of them, most likely in the morning, would cast off the equivalent of a wineglass," Stefansson wrote in *The Fat of the Land.*

Canned liver is usually easier to find — and more accessible in terms of taste, such as poultry liver (chicken, duck, goose) or baby animal liver (such as veal and lamb). In contrast, beef, goat, and pig liver all have a much stronger taste and some consider it absolutely unpalatable. Just one note: Food quality directly ties to flavour. Grass-fed ruminant liver, which is naturally raised, even from an older animal, will taste considerably better than conventionally raised beef liver.

Certain advantages of cod liver (and other fish livers) are their large quantities of Omega-3 fatty acids and iodine, whereas poultry livers tend to have higher concentrations of vitamin K2. And as with beef, the taste gets better when the animal has lived a natural life on the farm— not to mention the overall liver nutrient profile. Often, freshly slaughtered meat is much milder on taste. So if you get liver that hasn't been sitting in a freezer store for months, even people who don't like the flavour will be less disagreeable. Natural variation also exists in all the cases. For example, beef liver is higher in B vitamins, while goose liver is higher in vitamin K2 and duck liver has a lot of iron.

While finding a way to consume some form of liver pays off, those who simply cannot choke anything down can get (much) smaller amounts from eggs or some dairy. But the chickens have to be free-range really. And the milk must be non-pasteurized and originate from cows fed with grass. Otherwise, the content of Vitamin A is very difficult to know, and is likely to be negligible.

There is no natural vitamin A left in a store-bought carton of milk. However manufacturers also add synthetic vitamin A in the form of retinyl palmitate— which may be harmful to human liver. That is just another reason to stay away from conventional dairy production.

Since high quality variants of these foods are often difficult to accurately source, liver is always the best way to get there. Especially at the outset, as you can compensate for your (probable) past deficiency. Over time, when you replenish supplies with Vitamin A, you can do OK to get by on eggs, raw dairy and other animal fat fed with grass.

Each effort in the sourcing and preparation of food is important in any case. Canned cod liver and different pâtés are available, or even can be made at home. It's as easy as dumping some liver in a bowl and mixing it with some raw cream, raw butter, and raw honey. This is a super high, tasty, and approachable nutrient. It's like ice cream on the liver. Dip into it some slices of raw parmesan cheese (or some form of cracker that's healthier if you have to).

Of course you can just sauté or grill the liver on your own as well. It can be very bitter and astringent, as well as of low quality from animals that are raised conventionally.

That will be alleviated by buying grass-fed, especially younger animals. If you only have access to low-quality liver, soaking it in milk (or wine, or anything you can really think of) for 24 hours is a good option.

After marinating, I prefer to dry out the surface by leaving it on a rack in the refrigerator overnight, and then sear it in butter the next day. Eating it this way with generous salt and pepper, or with cheese bits or even some hot sauce on top, will make it easy to eat 100 grams or so a few days a week, which is enough to get the vitamin A you need.

I put liver on a wood fire, too, and it's an OK option but not really my favorite. Depending on how strict you are and what your dietary goals are, you can also use different types of meal to bread and fry it, although I don't think it's really necessary to marinate the liver properly and dry it out. The Eskimos liked boiling liver, and certain people ate it raw.

Personally, I've tried everything in the past— even swallowing raw liver.

So, if you're all just swallowing the liver to get your nutrition, then you can. It's just that there's more fun ways to go.

OMEGA-3 FATTY-ACIDS

The other fat-soluble vitamins are crucial as has already been said. But before I move on to those, I'd like to talk about another aspect of a healthy diet that has puzzled many people: Omega-3 fatty acids.

By now everyone knows they're significant. Over the past decade, perhaps no product has received more exposure than fish oil and its role in bringing us the Omega-3s we need. But even with all the recommendations, people remain misguided as to why they are so critical to consume. First off, many of these Omega fatty acids have to be obtained through diet, but they go far beyond just popping a few pills. Because you need to match the Omega-3 levels adequately with the other fats you eat, namely the Omega-6s that are massively over-consumed in the standard American diet, in addition to just having an allotted amount of milligrams per day.

While I don't want to over-complicate this, you need to learn some more granular details to get it right. For starters, three different types of Omega 3s actually exist: EPA (eicosapentaenoic acid), DHA (docosahexaenoic acid), and ALA (alpha-linolenic acid).

Our bread and butter are EPA and DHA— the two types that are present only in animal feed. That is what you need to focus every day on acquiring.

Such fatty acids mainly help regulate cellular inflammation (EPA) and preserve optimum brain health, structure of nerve cells and activity of the nerve cells (DHA). Although EPA produces beneficial chemicals called eicosanoids that are involved in anti-inflammatory processes, DHA must always be given priority as it is a brain necessity that requires such acids at a rate of about 4.6 mg per day.

DHA's role in early human development is important and its rates in breast milk vary from 0.06 to 1.4 per cent— a 20-fold variance!

As one real-world example, we might be able to look at the vascular properties of northern Canada's indigenous Inuit "Eskimos." Likely because of their high consumption of DHA and EPA, as chronicled by Weston Price in the early 1900s, their blood coagulated much slower, at about nine minutes, than the average of four minutes for people living in the US. This is due to platelet adhesivity, as well as fibrinogen accumulation in the blood. And when their blood flows so effortlessly, no wonder they had no heart disease to worry about!

The third type, ALA, is Omega-3 primarily found in plant foods, especially seed oils (usually marked as "vegetable oils") such as canola, soybean, maize, safflower, and palm oils. ALA can be processed in adipose tissue until ingested, and used for energy production.

There is a widespread belief that directly consuming the animal sources of Omega-3s is unnecessary since the body will transform ALA into EPA and DHA. But in a practical sense, that is more theory than fact. The conversion of ALA to EPA is low, usually less than 5 per cent, and in any trials, ALA intake has not been shown to increase blood levels of DHA.

Conversion rates will potentially be higher in a more theoretical sense. But this doesn't happen effectively in the presence of high levels of Omega-6— which are almost universal in modern U.S. diet (especially among vegetarians and vegans who often lack EPA and DHA).

This is because Omega-6 fatty acids fight for the Delta 6 Desaturase enzyme for conversion at multiple stages of its metabolism to DHA, without making it into a science textbook. And that process is significantly impaired when almost everyone consumes a high-Omega-6 diet.

Most indigenous groups are thought to have been completely free from heart disease along similar lines, and one factor suggested in this is the lack of seed oils and other highly processed modern food.

Finally, it should be remembered that high levels of Omega-6 can cause death of mitochondrial cells, and are generally a driving factor causing many diseases. Linoleic acid, a commonly consumed Omega-6 fatty acid, can cause necrotic cell death when produced in excessive quantities, whereas conjugated linoleic acid (an Omega-6 found in animal feeding stuffs) almost has the reverse effect.

What this and the rest of the knowledge, it shows us we need to keep the right balance between Omega-6s and Omega-3s — a ratio that has gotten out of whack over the past few decades.

According to a report from the Center for Genetics, Food, and Health in Washington, this ratio was possibly about 1 to 1 in ancestral times, while it has now risen to more than 15 to 1, or even higher. Western diets (especially in the United States) are low in Omega-3 fatty acids and have excessive amounts of Omega-6 fatty acids relative to the diet on which human beings have developed and their genetic patterns have been created," more and more evidence now suggests that uncontrolled levels of Omega-6s — and the resultant inflammation — are among the leading causes of the health crisis in our nation in the modern diet.

Because of this, Omega-3s are widely viewed as a pure supplement that will help lessen the damage much the same way that we are advised to eat blueberries and drink wines for their antioxidant properties.

In fact, people have been duped into thinking they can simply pop a fish oil pill every day and shield their hearts from all the damage done by the seed oils (and sugar) they cram down their throats every day.

The economy took advantage of that ignorance. It now pumps out billions of products filled with chemicals from the low-quality fish oil. So even if taking a small daily serving could do anything for you, it won't help if you're taking mass-produced pills that ignore the vital DHA and EPA to instead just pump you full of less-useful ALA. (These mass-market, low-quality pills are also often highly oxidized.) DHA and Omega-3s have to become a staple— not a supplement.

It is important to fill your diet with Omega-3s because, as noted, both DHA and EPA are essential to core bodily functions. The goal is not to hit some tiny milligram marker recommended by your doctor. What you have to do is get back the ratio of Omega-3s to Omega-6s in accordance with the natural feeding our ancestors have been doing for the last hundred thousand years.

This requires some homework and understanding of the different ratios in various foods. This is the reason why wild-caught salmon is so much more beneficial to your health, beyond pesticides and unsafe practices. Since ocean pollution can be very bad near the coast, farmed fish actually are one of the most dangerous foods to eat.

From a nutrient point of view, yes, farmed Atlantic salmon have more overall fat — and even more Omega-3s — as compared to wild-caught sockeye salmon. But it's chocked full of Omega-6s, too. Sockeye and other wild-caught varieties meanwhile have almost no Omega-6s. So it doesn't matter that their total content on Omega-3 is also less. There's just a much better nutrient profile.

You boost your body ratios by eating sockeye. And while we're going to detail all of this later, that's the same reason why eating conventionally raised chicken and pork doesn't make you favourites. Wild fowl and feral hogs do have good Omega ratios for human consumption. But because these animals ' feedlot-raised varieties eat soy and corn rather than their natural feeding diet (which may include acorns and insects), their fat stores become laden with the same Omega-6s we are trying to avoid. These animals just like you do, become what they eat.

Fixing the Omega ratio involves two practical steps: the Omega-3s (in DHA and EPA form) and taking out the Omega-6s.

You can't do that with a tablet, or even by buying a farm-raised salmon filet once a week. That requires a concerted effort.

Ultimately, fixing Omega ratios is something that will inherently happen over time when seed oils are removed and foods of higher quality begin to make up the majority of your diet. But fish does help, and high-quality fish oils will accelerate that process. This is important because an imbalanced Omega-3 to Omega-6 ratio will increase oxidative stress— a driving force for most diseases.

OMEGA-3: SOURCES & PREPARATION - There are two reasons we need to concentrate on getting DHA, more so than EPA and ALA. First, when it comes to human metabolism, the others are not as equally important. However, second, in most instances EPA comes naturally with high-DHA products. This is good news that simplifies everything: you'll be good to go if you eat foods loaded in DHA.

How do we get this done? Seafood — and plenty of it. The fattier the fish, the better (the most common being the wild-caught salmon). On a per-calorie basis, fish eggs (look for salmon roe) are even higher in DHA, making them one of the leading true "superfoods" out there. Normal chicken eggs are possibly the most available source of DHA, but due to grain feeding they also have a high content of Omega-6. As much as wild-caught vs. farm-raised fish, if they are truly free-range, they are only a high-level choice.

One great alternative is animal brain intake, which is very high in DHA. Unlike fish eggs, their DHA is in the form of phospholipids, which our own brains are said to have more exposure to. I eat them quite often but most people are not going to go to such great lengths for their food, understandably.

Yet pan-seared lamb or veal brains are definitely worth a try— if you can find and treat them.

Some people believe fish is very tricky to cook when it comes to preparation. And without any experience, that can be. But even experienced cooks usually learn quickly that just baking a salmon filet with salt, pepper, and butter in an oven for 15 minutes can be a delicious meal. Even better is to sauté a skin-down filet with some oil in a saucepan. It may take a few tries, but you'll soon learn that you can cook it as rare or as well done as you like, and get away with the wonderfully crispy skin and the translucent pink flesh that chefs around the world would envy you.

Personally I enjoy fish eggs as often as I can find them for ease and the best DHA density per calorie. While the actual caviar is prohibitively expensive, salmon roe (or other forms of roe) is often available in cities or Asian markets from local fish suppliers. All you need is a few teaspoons in a day a couple of times a week to get the DHA you need (when paired with a broader diet of other high-quality animal foods).

Sashimi is another favorite of mine, but eating it out can be expensive and it is a bit tedious to prepare yourself. Canned fish can also work and at a budget, things like sardines and anchovies are great for anyone.

VITAMIN K2

Next to our list is a nutrient which most people completely overlook when thinking about their health: vitamin K2. This vitamin is thought to play a role in skeletal health, in the form of MK7. But its sister variant, MK4, is much more relevant, and can be transformed into any other forms we need. Animal foods contain mainly MK4, which also plays a key role in preventing the build-up of calcium in organs and tissues, including the arteries.

Besides these types, there is vitamin K1, which is commonly found in plant foods and cannot be converted effectively to Vitamin K2 in animal foods. Then there are a few other types (MK8, MK9, MK10, and MK11) that occur in various animal feeds. Yet vitamin K2 is probably the group's most important and sadly it's also the hardest vitamin to get into our diets.

The factor that makes vitamin K2 so important is it stimulates MGP (Matrix Gla Protein), which enables proper transport of calcium within the body. And outside of vascular health, the series of "menaquinones" collectively known as Vitamin K2 are linked to exercise performance, sexual health, insulin sensitivity reduction and, some studies show cancer-protection.

That all sounds important. But what makes K2 stronger than some of the other vitamins? Well, it's not that this is necessarily more important in general. It's just that a lot of people just don't get enough of it. And this is easy to fix, because it's largely because they don't value Vitamin K2 and ignore the few good sources that exist.

Unlike the B vitamins most people simply accumulate in their diet by accident, you need to look for Vitamin K2, largely in the form of fermented foods or high-quality eggs. All animal foods of high quality contain small amounts of Vitamin K2. Liver and eggs are likewise decent sources. Nevertheless, the secret is fermented foods such as cheese.

You must also ensure that your gut health remains good, so that the bacteria that live there can continue to produce at least some of what we need. Yes, the bugs inside your intestines do some of the work here for you as long as you don't kill your bowels with a bad diet and antibiotics.

"The absorption and transportation of Vitamin K produced by gut bacteria is little known, but research shows that substantial amounts... are present in the large intestine," according to the National Institute of Health (NIH). "Although the amount of Vitamin K obtained by the body in this manner is unclear, experts believe that these menaquinones satisfy at least some of the body's requirements.

VITAMIN K2: SOURCES AND PREPARATION

Vitamin K2, like Vitamin A, is to some extent contained in many animal feeds depending on the quality of the pasture. This is because the chlorophyll in the grass in the animal's tissue turns into vitamin K2. And this initial amount will then rise by fermentation.

As far as sources of higher volume are concerned, eggs are really the only food that contains any substantial amount of vitamin K2 you would be cooking for. However, as with DHA, you will have much better results in this department by heading out with truly free-range eggs laid by birds consuming their natural diet outside.

The other good source comes as fermented food. This is because Vitamin K2 is gradually evolving as the products age as bacteria play a role in producing that essential vitamin, as they do in your stomach.

The obvious choice is bacon. But you won't get that nutrient from the bulk of the "cheese" that you'll find in a supermarket. You need to look for "raw" grass-fed cheese (meaning it's made from unpasteurized milk).

Various European types tend to fill the bill. Some good choices include Italy's Parmigiano-Reggiano, Switzerland's gruyere-like variety L'Étivaz, and Auvergne Bleu, among other famous French blue cheeses. As a rule, if a cheese has received a formal protective certification from its local jurisdiction, this ensures that it is produced the traditional way and will preserve much of its natural nutrient content. The Swiss cheese is probably the best overall, followed by France and Spain. Origin nation does not guarantee quality, but these are usually better on average and each has specific cheeses which are always made in a more traditional, nutritious manner.

In the United States, at local farms that sell raw cheese or aged types (which can be legally made from unpasteurized dairy) in specialty stores (or even Whole Foods these days), you'll have the best luck. Also, cheeses made from goat and sheep's milk tend to be fed grass more frequently than those coming from cow's milk because these animals usually live outside, at least for most of their lives, rather than in a feedlot.

Although the number of sources for Vitamin K2 is somewhat limited, the good news is that all of this is relatively palatable and easy to consume. Just good, aged cheeses and fermented meats are all you need. And, as already described, maintaining a healthy intestine will also help.

VITAMIN D3

Vitamin D3 is the last of four essential nutrients listed here.

Unlike Vitamin A, hundreds of genes are precursors for cell differentiation and gene expression. It means the value of it often flies under the radar, with most people only recognizing its role in the metabolism of calcium.

It is definitely important for bone homeostasis, given its association with hormones that signal the absorption and release of calcium. And through decades of Got Milk and It Does a Body Good ads, you've certainly heard of milk being fortified with Vitamin D to support good health (after most of the real nutrients are destroyed by pasteurization).

But this is only a part of the story, as we can see in other key areas. Vitamin D3 is needed to produce many hormones and can be associated with many common human diseases that have low levels. Also cancer therapy has proven to be effective. Even the doctors seem to catch on. We conduct further tests and regularly encourage patients to begin supplementing them. Even though their aim is generally to avoid bone loss, a positive development has been the more widespread understanding of the value of Vitamin D.

Today, there are two main problems stopping many citizens from reaching adequate levels. The first is the biggest reason: the sun scares us. People have always obtained the majority of their Vitamin D3 simply by living outdoors and spending a lot of time there. Our bodies contain a "zoosterol" substance called 7-Dehydrocholesterol that, in the presence of UV light, can be photochemically transformed into Vitamin D3.

They used to be in the sun most of the day, throughout history. Our "services" were simply food production, and hunting or harvesting crops outside was the only way to procure food.

For anyone living near the equator, having enough UV light certainly never was a concern. But for the majority of the year, far northern and southern latitudes may have had lower UV indexes, meaning that people native to these areas would have had to eat more Vitamin D3 from food sources.

This brings us to the second problem these modern people have when it comes to achieving adequate levels: quality of food. Only people living in areas like Russia could get enough Vitamin D3 from food, thousands of years ago. This is because other species transform UV rays into Vitamin D3 just as other humans do. Before the last few decades, wild game, fish, and even livestock would spend the entire day outdoors and collect a substantial amount.

What humans needed to do was feed these animals a sufficiently large quantity— which they were already doing just to get energy calories — and they'd be set.

Even if you look at more modern Russian indigenous groups, their levels of Vitamin D3 may range from around 40 ng / ml to 67 ng / ml (nanograms / milliliter) — triple the amount most people have today.

The 40 ng / ml level is a critical threshold, because this is when your body will have more than enough for all current needs and start winter storage of Vitamin D3.

Anything lower than that and at any time the sun's rays are sparse you run essentially on empty. Depending on who you are asking, from 40 ng / ml to 80 ng / ml is considered healthy anywhere. The National Institute of Health considers 12 ng / ml or less to be a "deficiency," but notes that even between 12 ng / ml and 20 ng / ml is "generally considered inadequate in healthy individuals for bone and overall health."

What does that really mean with everything that's been said? Although checking for levels of Vitamin D3 is a good idea, those levels of blood are not something you can regularly monitor. And, sadly, here we have another problem relating to the RDA.

To people 70 years old or younger, the RDA recommendation of 600 IU (international units) per day is actually based on a statistical fallacy.

Shockingly, the real Vitamin D3 RDA should have always been at least 10 times that figure— something about which more and more scientists have come to sound the alarm.

In particular, in 2015, studies at UC San Diego and Creighton University led to the publication of a letter in the journal Nutrients advocating a correction. "We call on the IOM and all public health authorities concerned to provide the public with accurate nutritional information to designate, as the RDA, a value of approximately 7,000 IU per day from all sources," wrote Dr Robert Heaney of Creighton University.

One fuckin' error, huh? Another research in Nutrients ("A Statistical Error in Vitamin D's Estimated Recommended Dietary Allowance") found that the right estimate could even be as high as 8,895 IU per day.

But this mistake has long been recognized by many, based on the knowledge that the body can contain more than 40,000 IU per day. Finally, now the world of nutrition is beginning to come around.

This is a great metaphor for all areas of our modern diet, in a sad way. After decades of denial, and moving in the wrong direction, some people are finally beginning to recognize how everything is out of whack.

VITAMIN D3: SOURCES & PREPARATION

It's helpful to know certain numbers. But for the average person, to only one level. If our goal is 60 ng / ml or 7,000(+) IU / day, how do we get that much Vitamin D3?

Getting some sun is the best way to go and then you can rely on high-quality food sources, supplements or even tanning beds as well. Now more than ever, people are worried about skin cancer and there is reason to be cautious.

But especially if the rest of your nutrition is on spot— and you get enough Vitamin A, which works somewhat in conjunction with vitamin D3 — you're probably more worried than you need to be.

Always consult with your doctor, but usually getting more sun will do more good than harm even when you're factoring in the level of potential risk.

The amount of sun exposure you need depends on different factors, too. You need to grasp the UV level at different times of year and in different geographies.

Even in a relatively sunny place like Los Angeles, for instance, during the winter, you wouldn't get nearly as much Vitamin D3 from the sun because of the Earth's tilt. The sunlight is composed of two types of UV light, called UVB and UVA rays, without becoming too scientific. This is actually about 95 per cent UVA and 5 per cent UVB during much of the day in the summer in most areas. And conversion of Vitamin D3 is the product of the UVB rays. But sunbathing from 8 a.m. to 10 a.m. might not do you a lot of good actually.

Nevertheless, the UVB level may be as high as 20 per cent during the "max UV" hours from about 11 am to 1 pm. So while you want to be vigilant and consider how your individual skin reacts to a clear day at peak UV, in a shorter exposure midday period, you can get a lot more bang for your buck. (And as noted, that depends greatly on your latitude. People in Maine, Florida and Ecuador also experience very different levels of UVB at different times of the year and at different times of the day.)

Vitamin D3 conversion may also vary depending on skin colour. In warmer months, when you are outside at peak UV, the amount of absorption between people with pale white skin, olive skin, brown skin and black skin can differ dramatically. Over the course of the season, our ancestors would have slowly adjusted to the sun so when the scorching summer heat arrived their skin was ready for it.

There are also rising sun exposure returns — for any person in any location— related to how often you are outside as well as how your skin is increasingly tanning. As a rule, being out in the sun for one hour per day at peak UV is usually better than being out seven hours once a week. Your skin can only absorb so much per day, so spreading it out frequently is ideal. This also helps keep you from overdoing it and causing sunburn.

Tanning beds are an alternative for people living in Minneapolis in January — and, indeed, just anyone at any time who very often can't get outside midday. Nonetheless, the one thing to keep an eye on is the UVA / UVB ratio.

With regard to this ratio, many tanning beds fall in line with the sun but, as both tan your skin equally well, but some have very low levels of UVB.

This can be as low as or less than 1 per cent. So be sure to ask or look up the tanning bed model to ensure it gives you the necessary UVB rays that are essential for the production of Vitamin D3. (Tanning beds also have electromagnetic fields, EMF, problems that should be known before risking this option.) As with our ancestors in Russia and Norway, food is also a good source of Vitamin D3 for people today. The only drawback is that feedlot cows and conventionally raised chicken typically spend a great deal of their lives indoors. So, besides all the other aforementioned problems that this causes nutritionally, they also don't contain the natural levels of wild game or grass-fed, free-grazing beef Vitamin D3. The same applies to traditional dairy and eggs, although these are often fortified with Vitamin D3 (although the other nutritional downsides ultimately make them not worth consuming).

For that reason, fatty fish such as mackerel, herring, sardines, and anchovies are the best easily accessible and affordable sources for most people. Fish roe is fantastic too. Wild-caught is always better for all seafood, while farmed fish generally provide more nutrients than farmed animals on the ground.

Ultimately, if you wonder if an animal source is going to be high or low in Vitamin D3, ask yourself this: Did it live in the sun for most of its lifetime? If the answer is "no," there won't be much Vitamin D3 in its meat, fat, and byproducts. Making sense?

Supplementation is another issue to remember. For anyone and particularly for the Minneapolis college student in January who can't afford grass-fed beef or tanning beds this can be beneficial. Vitamin D3 supplements are relatively cheap, though you should try to find a brand that's well known.

Make sure to keep this in mind if you go with drops or pills: Vitamin D3 in supplement form is metabolized differently than it is from the sun. It is absorbed much quicker. So you have to make certain precautions. Rather than taking a large amount of Vitamin D3 drops or pills all at once, spreading it out over the course of the day is ideal. (Many people think it is better to take it better earlier in the day, as it can often cause sleep problems if taken too late at night.) Eventually, there is one more consideration: Vitamin D3 also goes hand in hand with Vitamin K2, which binds to calcium and moves it into and out of different tissues. Without Vitamin K2, we probably wouldn't have had Vitamin D3 in nature. Chances are, if we were in the sun for a long time, we would be eating better animal foods containing Vitamin K2. It is something you need to keep in mind in modern times when supplementation is commonplace (though following the ancestral indigenous diet means you will always prioritize both).

Vitamin D3 can be loaded at the outset when it comes to fixing past deficiencies. But the need to maintain synergy with the nutrients can make things here difficult. When you can quickly get massive amounts of Vitamin A and Vitamin D3 from the liver and supplements, it's hard to balance all of this with normal levels of Vitamin K2 (as well as other minerals).

For some people, loading up large amounts of Vitamin D3 may initially work.

But those nutrients are not an experiment in science at high school. When they become unbalanced, their chief feature (calcium metabolism) can be increased rapidly enough to cause problems.

I don't want to start to scare people off taking higher amounts.

Therefore, I always suggest that you get a blood test. This will let you know if in fact you are seriously deficient. If so, it could mean that loading up will be more positive than the potential downside of discarding your synergy with nutrients. Otherwise, you might be better off sticking to normal recommended levels of consumption.

THE ROLE OF FAT- I want to analyze fat first in general before we move on to the other micronutrients you need. Do not make a mistake: Fat is a macronutrient— not one of the micronutrients we are talking about here. Nevertheless, understanding its role in the metabolism and overall optimum human health is essential.

All fat soluble vitamins include Vitamin A, Vitamin K2, and Vitamin D3. There it is in the name right there. Your diet needs enough fat to do its job for those nutrients.

First-nation Alaskans on carnivorous diets used to get about 80% of their calories from fat and 20% from protein. This is a simplistic response to macronutrient ratios, since the sheer variety of foods in all native diets resulted in high variance depending on the geographic location. But they had adequate nutrition as long as the indigenous group received 45 percent -65 percent of their total calories from animal foods.

For some reason, fat-soluble vitamins are called so. Instead of muscle meat, they are contained in the fatty parts of the animal, as well as in the organs.

We are therefore, increasing the overall nutrient density in the diet by consuming most of our calories from high-fat animal foods (including fatty muscle meats such as ribeye steak) (provided these are high-quality foods).

Another important reason to concentrate on fat consumption is what it does with a view to reducing the overall volume of food. Let us take a look at one case. If you eat half a pound of fat and one pound of protein instead of three pounds of lean protein, you can get the same number of calories in your stomach without causing so much digestive stress and bulk. That's pretty good! It means less work for your enzymes in the liver, lungs and digestive tract when having the same amount of nutrients (and in most cases even more).

We'll talk more about this in later chapters, but the more efficient your digestive system becomes, the less you'll experience inflammation and the better you feel.

And historically, the most important element of fat in ancient times was always mere survival. It was — and is — the fuel our bodies can use the easiest, and this is a major reason why people don't see success in diets that are purely high in protein, and low in both carbs and fat.

Yes, the body can make use of protein energy— but not almost as efficiently as it can from fats. (The same applies to a lesser extent to carbohydrates, because certain starches and sugars can stress certain organs and digestive enzymes much more than fat digestion.) Protein is of course necessary for the growth of muscle cells. But it's really a demand-driven need in the big picture and this depends on the lean body mass of the consumer. Because I used to be heavily involved in bodybuilding, I still hold about 20 pounds more muscle mass than an untrained person even now.

This means my body's protein requirement is significant, just to maintain my current physique. So instead of eating 80 percent of my calories from a source of energy (fat), my consumption may be more skewed towards carbohydrates, ranging about 60 percent-70 percent of calories from fat and the remainder from protein for anywhere.

That might not be the ratio you need personally. So this is something you can turn in over time, and you don't have to worry too much at the beginning. Generally speaking, you should be prepared to increase your fat consumption significantly compared to your previous eating habits and cut the carbs almost completely. The important part is not to get scared of fat. You need it and you want to consume one ton of it! Because without it you'll not only lack energy, but the fat-soluble vitamins won't get into the area they need to work best.

MONTHLY NUTRIENT REQUIREMENTS

Before we move on there's one more thing to address: "How much? "What kind of intake do you need from Vitamins A, K2, D3, and Omega-3s?

Now you should understand why the RDAs and DRIs aren't always appropriate. You can look at these to get a sense of what the results appear to look like, but sticking with that diet will usually work itself out over time.

If the food you eat is of high quality and your macronutrient ratios are correct, you don't have to worry about meeting the needs for vitamins and minerals. They'll be done because ultimately the food you eat has the right amounts. The best way to figure out how much nutrition you need is based on the fat ratios our indigenous ancestors used: 80 percent fat and 20 percent protein combined with an actual animal's organ-to-muscle-to-fat ratios.

Think of it like this: Eating 50 pounds of meat and 15 pounds of fat in a month would be the equivalent yield of perhaps one large sheep or goat. When we look at the size of the liver's organ tissue, this would possibly be anywhere from three to four pounds. One-and - a-half pounds of liver per 30 pounds of meat yield would be a conservative estimate.

This same analogy can be made to all of the animal's other organs, from the liver to the lungs to the spleen, to the adrenal glands, testicles, and on and on and on. We achieve a total nutrient profile by eating any part of the animal in ideal ratios. This is what we, in fact, would have done.

That gets more difficult when we don't want to eat tail to nose. While I personally take it to the extreme, I know it is a little bit much to ask you to eat lungs. And we don't necessarily need to do so in a modern society. There's a lot of liver to go around.

We should actually try to think about all the organs' total nutrient profile, and look into alternatives. A hunter-gatherer would have earned DHA from the brains, but, actually, instead you can eat only fatty fish or eggs.

Maybe you prefer beef liver to chicken liver. If so, eat it from a cow just eat more of those smaller varieties than one large one.

In general, you want to adhere to the guidelines, consider the vitamins and nutrients you need, and stay away from the negative foods. But you needn't overcomplicate things as well.

We know that nearly all known indigenous groups obtained most of their calories from animal food. However, we also know that the exact quantities varied quite a bit according to culture and geographic region. Although we don't know exactly how their health might have changed due to dietary choices, physical presence and statute was one widely observed difference between groups consuming around two-thirds of their calories from animal foods and groups consuming up to 85 percent from animal food.

We've heard stories, for example, that the Mongols are very tall and strong in Central Asia. When they invaded the Germanic parts of Europe, the Roman troops often said these men were very tall and physically imposing. Captains of the Age of Exploration who landed in North America were often surprised by how good the native population was at hunting, particularly in their stamina and ability to chase game down. Throughout time there have always been fascinating stories about the physical condition of indigenous communities, though just anecdotes.

We don't always have to be incredibly precise about everything.

Because, for one, we have better access than our ancestors to all those sources. Getting adequate fat should be simple, as well as getting all the liver that we can stomach. As long as replenish your stores every week, you'll be fine.

Second, note these are vitamins which are fat-soluble. You're going to hold some inside your body. You'll be doing pretty good as long as you eat just a few hundred grams of liver every week, eat some quality cheese, eat something out of the ocean, and get some sunshine. Then add in some free-range eggs to be safe — together with an overall diet based on high-quality animal foods, including seafood. There are optimal eating habits to strive for but you don't need to make things over-complicated to start getting real, natural nutrition into your diet.

However, you also need to consider past deficits. If you've eaten a SAD diet forever, there's likely to be a significant lack in all four of these areas. You shouldn't try overnight to compensate for decades of poor nutrition. Don't start filling in like a madman.

But that does mean you can pay extra attention rather than slip up. I've eaten this way for years. If I get no liver in my system for two weeks, it's not going to be the end of the world. Nevertheless you need to make up for lost time.

Act diligently in all aspects, so you can step forward as quickly as possible on your path towards better health.

With time, you'll begin to understand everything involved— including how your body responds — and start dialing everything in much more accurately. You will compensate for shortages, start repairing your Omega ratios and get all the vitamins and minerals in the right balance.

It'll take quite some time. But you'll be far ahead of most people and well on your way to optimal health just by beginning on this road and knowing the principles discussed so far.

CHAPTER 3: BENEFITS OF THE CARNIVORE DIET

Let's begin with the commonly reported benefits of eating a carnivorous diet. Your mileage may vary yet again. Everyone does not always see these results. Diet is only one of so many factors in determining wellbeing, although it plays a huge role.

There are various benefits you'll reap when you properly adopt this meat-based diet.

Weight loss-Many people doubt it when they hear that a diet based solely on meat will help them lose weight or even improve their health; but, when you know more about it, you can understand exactly why it is real. Let me tell you, this diet allows you to abstain from carbohydrate consumption. If the intake of carbohydrates is low, the blood sugar levels are the same, and this prevents spikes of insulin.

This, in turn, will prevent the deposit of calories in your body in the form of fats that then lead to weight gain or even obesity. Reducing dietary carbohydrates often helps you avoid unnecessary calorie consumption, and also decreases unhealthy eating. During your daily activities your body just needs as many calories as it takes for energy.

If you don't burn much but eat more calories, it's just going to get accumulated in your body. For this reason the Carnivore Diet carbohydrate deficiency will help you lose weight. Actually, it helps to increase the amount of proteins and fats you eat, and this will help relieve your long-term appetite. It'll also get rid of excessive cravings or hunger pangs. Despite knowing it, a lot of people gain weight as they eat absent-mindedly.

The Carnivore Diet also helps to reduce this, because you won't feel hungry all the time and will eat more attentively when you're hungry. When you think about it, the foods we eat while watching TV, reading a book, and so on are typically junk foods we just keep shoving into our mouths. If the diet is limited to meat, snacking on a steak or any other form of meat is hardly likely to continue.

Over time, it will help you distinguish between real hunger and psychological hunger when you adopt the diet. On this diet, you can't reach out for a bag of chips at any time you want, so your calorie intake is reduced even without any calorie counting. Reducing the intake of carbohydrates often forces the body into ketosis, as in the Ketogenic diet. Then your body burns fat for energy, and helps you lose more weight.

If you want a summary of how this diet makes you lose weight, consider the following. This makes you eat more fat, and drink more water. It limits the food types you can eat, and also reduces oil, sugar, and flour. Instead, you will eat food which is higher in volume, and this will result in better chewing and digestion aid. The diet will thus help with weight loss.

Improved skin including skin tag clearing, acne clearing, eliminating eczema, and anti-aging effects are seen on the skin as anti-inflammatory foods replace the dietary carbohydrates.

The cravings for carbohydrates finally disappear. It usually happens after a transition period of 1-3 weeks, when the person comes from a diet rich in carbohydrates. They're already more fat-adapted for people coming from a keto diet and carb cravings can be reduced much quicker. Once the cravings have disappeared it will stick. Plop a piece of cake in front of one of these people, and they don't have any problem passing on it. There's just not desire. I'd rather have a ribeye, in my case.

Loss of fat.

There are countless testimonials that show people losing weight on a Carnivore Diet. Want to really get inspired for thirty minutes? Visit MeatHeals.com and browse the images of a Carnivore Diet before and after. People are losing weight, and gaining strength. It's effortless because they're pleased with the diet (the meat is delicious after all), and the cravings are regulated or non-existent.

Some people can gain weight, on the flipside... Well, in a good way. If a person comes to the diet with malnutrition, some weight can be gained, perhaps only temporarily, as the body reconstitutes and changes from a carbohydrate-driven metabolism to a fat-adapted one. Hence, some people argue that the Carnivore Diet is not a "weight-loss" diet, but rather that it burns fat and promotes muscle growth, making it an "improved body composition" diet in general.

Testosterone increased in men

According to a study in the American Journal of Clinical Nutrition, men who ate a diet high in fat, and low in fiber for 10 weeks saw a 13 percent increase in testosterone higher than the low-fat, high-fiber group. Consuming more fat in your diet will naturally help boost your body's level of testosterone. Studies have demonstrated this by comparing men who had a high-fat diet with men with low-fat diets. The Carnivore Diet is therefore advantageous for men to increase healthy levels of testosterone, as well as to reduce the incidence of pain and migraine headaches.

Reduced joint aches and bruising with reduced inflammation.

Improvement of allergies

It refers to both food allergies (because of the Carnivore Diet's eliminative aspect and the cure that happens) and seasonal allergies.

More libido.

Straightforwardness.

It is a simple diet, easy to get started and easy to maintain. There are no complicated recipes to follow and you'll spend far less time in the grocery store and kitchen.

Improved digestion, and less time trying to poop in the bathroom for long periods of time. Many people report dramatic improvements in their digestive disorders (life-change), as a result of no longer consuming unpleasant foods. If your diet is unhealthy, the digestive system is a major cause of concern. Most people argue that high amounts of fiber in the diet are important for digestive health; this is not necessarily true though. A study showed you could support the digestive system by growing fiber. Hence, the Carnivore Diet can help treat constipation, improve bowel movements and also reduce bloating or gas.

Quality improved with many studies requiring less quality.

Cognition and focus improved.

Gains in power, and increased recovery time. Athletes have reported strength gains and faster recovery from protein-rich and nutrient-rich foods such as beef, and a reduction of inflammatory foods.

Facilitating muscle maintenance.

When eating carnivore, some people have reduced the strength of exercises, but notice they are able to maintain muscle and have great definition. (I found personal joy in this one as we travel abroad without access to a gym.) Feeling mentally better, with a dramatic improvement in mood. People are reporting that depression is going away. They're motivated and they feel strong and happy. Trust in abundance as they perform exceptionally.

Cardiovascular health

A few decades ago, meat and even eggs started to be blamed for the growing occurrence of heart disease, but we know it isn't that simple. Processed meat is generally linked to heart disease when it comes to meat and not red meat. You should pay attention not only to the cholesterol in foods, but also to the amount of saturated fat in them. Eating too much processed foods or carbohydrates can cause your body to increase its LDL level. LDL is the bad cholesterol that needs to be lowered in your body, while HDL is the good cholesterol that will protect your core. When the LDL levels increase, it negatively affects your cardiovascular health; however, you will increase the HDL levels on the Carnivore Diet and thus improve your heart condition.

Reduction of inflammation

In case of an inflammation in your body, your liver will produce something called C-reactive proteins or CRP. The level of this CRP indicates how much inflammation your body is experiencing. It is a misconception that foods derived from animals are causing inflammation. Reducing plant-sourced food intake would reduce the amount of inflammation that is suggested by high levels of CRP. You should take note of any specific plant foods in your body that cause inflammation and take care to cut those out of your diet. A meat-based diet will therefore help to reduce inflammation, and this will help to reduce discomfort in the joints or from arthritis.

Better oral health

Sugar impacts your oral health very unhealthily. It is one of the principal causes of cavities and also causes an imbalance in mouth pH levels. The Carnivore Diet cuts sugar out of your diet, and this helps restore a healthy pH. It will also prevent the breeding of bacteria in your mouth and the cause of any infections or decay in your teeth. There is also a lot of people suffering from gum disease and the Carnivore Diet helps control it and prevent it over time.

Improved eyesight

This may be questionable, but trust us when we say that sugar also has a very bad effect on your eyesight. Eliminating sugar from your diet also reduces the levels in your body. This then reduces the risk of cataracts and helps maintain healthy eyes.

THE EFFECT OF CARNIVORE DIET ON DIGESTION

Your digestive system plays a significant part in your body. Your diet, in effect, has a big impact on your digestion. That is why it's important to pay due attention to the impact on your digestion from the different foods you eat. Every system within your body is interlinked, and in other respects, a problem with one will also cause health problems. This segment should help you understand how the Carnivore Diet affects the digestive system.

Every healthy gut has a few kilograms of microbes within it. These include about a thousand different species of bacteria, and your digestive health will be affected by these microbes. Bacteria are not always bad. Some are in the digestive process naturally in your stomach and are essential for good health in the gut. They help your body use nutrients from the digested food. Neither the small intestine nor the stomach can ingest any type of food. The microbes come in at this point, and do it for them. Hence, supporting good microbe health in your gut is necessary. That will be decided by the foods you eat. In that, certain foods will help, and others will cause a negative reaction.

Sugar and processed food are not healthy for your digestive system. That's why the Carnivore Diet requires you to eliminate any such foods and focus on healthy foods based on fat and meat. Sugars and processed foods will cause the growth of unwanted bacteria in your gut. That will create an imbalance in your intestine in a healthy microbiome environment. This affects the digestive system and food is not digested in an appropriate manner. All the sugars, artificial sweeteners and ingredients in processed food are harming the good bacteria in your gut. That's why, if you want the probiotic bacteria to survive in your digestive system while removing harmful bacteria, the bad substances need to be eliminated.

In an unhealthy digestive system a leaky gut can be another concern. The Carnivore Diet also helps prevent this from happening and restores health. Not every substance in the foods you eat is good for your body. The good bacteria and healthy gut ensure they stay inside the gastrointestinal tract as they act as a barrier. The barrier is also not effective when your gut lining isn't in a healthy condition. It means the harmful substances will exit the gastrointestinal tract and enter the bloodstream. That can be a very risky body condition. Not only does harmful bacteria get into the bloodstream but also food particles and toxins. That is why it is important to pay attention to the health of the gut so as to maintain a healthy barrier.

A leaky gut can show adverse effects on different aspects of your body. That includes your skin, your hormones and your brain. You may wonder how the Carnivore Diet helps to prevent this. Therefore, dietary restriction plays an important role. Grains, and legumes can cause the barrier to weaken. The gluten in these foods may be a significant cause of autoimmune disorders.

There is a protein molecule called Zonulin which is activated by grain gluten. This molecule of protein breaks the bonds between the cells inside the intestinal walls and the gut lining. The lectins and phytic acids contained in these foods also weaken the barrier and are therefore detrimental to gut health. Such foods can also lead to leaky gut syndrome, which is a very unhealthy digestive disorder you need to avoid. The Carnivore Diet does not contain any of these grains or legumes, therefore it does not harm the gut lining. Instead, dietary fats will help release proteins that will reinforce the gut by decreasing inflammation.

The modern Western diet in terms of healthy dietary fats is sadly lacking. People have reduced their fat intake as much as possible as they believe it is the culprit behind weight gain and other health problems. The reality is that the cause is carbohydrates, and not the healthy fats. Instead, those carbs should be eliminated, and this is helped by the Carnivore Diet. You are encouraged to eat foods that have plenty of dietary fat like beef and dairy products instead.

Eating grass-fed meat along with seafood will provide you with a safe regular supply of omega 3 fatty acids. These are healthy and increase the bacteria diversity which is essential for proper digestion. This in-stomach microbiome unit is quite like a small ecosystem on its own and diversity is always a good way to evolve. The healthier the fats are your diet contains, the more diverse it will be, and hence the better for your health.

The toxic Western diet and lifestyle have exacerbated almost all of the health problems experienced by the past few generations. The way we cook, the way we all live has a negative effect on us and therefore, induces illness. The food in the modern diet is full of GMOs, pesticides, chemicals, additives, and so on, and this damages your intestines in general. You will improve the health of the digestive system by switching to the basic eating method followed by our ancestors. The more that you eat processed food, the worse it gets. The Carnivore Diet will help prevent this kind of unhealthy condition.

If you're worried about the diet's lack of fiber, you shouldn't be. It has been said to most of us that fiber is essential to a healthy digestive system and daily bowel movements. This factor is missing from the Carnivore Diet; however, fiber isn't as important as it is made out to be. Instead of protein, the food's good fat can help regulate your intestines.

Such dietary fats stimulate the body's waste disposal process. You might find it's less popular than usual, but that's natural. The carnivorous diet itself is the explanation for this. The body simply doesn't need to get rid of as much waste as the usual diet does. It's true that fiber is important to some people because of their particular genetic makeup, but a high fiber diet isn't necessary for everyone.

You have to know that in some way or the other, every system in the body is interlinked, so the digestive system is also connected to the brain. The heart in your body functions like a new brain. That's why when you have to make some decisions, people say, "Go with your gut." There's a lot of research that says the gut and mind are very much connected. Your gut is strongly connected to your emotions even if you haven't thought about it before. Have you noticed how your stomach seems to feel achy when you're scared or nervous, or how sometimes there's a feeling like butterflies moving?

This is why the intestines have so many sayings about them. That too is backed by scientific reasoning. In the gut there is the enteric nervous system, or ENS. This ENS controls the secretions within the gastrointestinal tract and the blood flow. You can sense what's happening in your gut because of this device. This is why the stomach has so much control over the body's digestion.

Even this is linked to the workings of your stomach when you feel tension. Do you know about the ability to fight or to fly? In humans this is an instinct which helps them to protect themselves. The instinct is responsible for regulating the body's level of cortisol. The body normally functions when stress is not present. But when you experience stress, this fight or flight emotion is experienced by the body too.

The human body is unable to distinguish between physical and psychological stress. You are at high risk of chronic inflammation if you are someone who is dealing with chronic stress or anxiety. It will respond in case of stress the same way your body reacts if there is an infection. If you want to prevent the damage from inflammation on your system, it is important to try and alleviate such stress from your everyday life. Pay attention to the relationship between the mind and the gut. The body has a way to let you know when it is in distress, so you can make an effort to look after it. If you eat a healthy diet such as the Carnivore Diet, it will improve the health of your gut and also ensure good mental health.

THE EFFECT OF CARNIVORE DIET ON CHOLESTEROL

Eating meat, butter or even eggs is one of the main causes of elevated levels of bad cholesterol. You're going to hear a lot of so-called weight gurus telling you to stop eating any of these if you want to lose weight or get better. You probably doubt the validity of us claiming that a diet that is rich in these foods will have no effect on your health in any way, particularly in terms of alcohol. It could make you feel as if we said eating a lot of junk food will not make you fat. But on a frank note, the two are not similar in any way.

Cholesterol itself has a lot of misconceptions to it. In this segment, we'll try to explain more about how your diet affects your cholesterol levels and whether or not you should be concerned. But you have to keep an open mind before you do this, and let go of the misconceptions you already have. Only then will you understand how it works and why you get healthy on the Carnivore Diet.

Most of what we know about cholesterol is not true, and is based on unreasonable statements made by some people who don't understand anything better themselves. Cholesterol is a wax-like substance which humans and animals produce. No other living form produces cholesterol; so, it is free of all plant sources. Much research has demonstrated that people with clogged arteries are more likely to suffer from cardiovascular health problems. There is a direct connection between the arteries and your heart and this affects your health.

The more your arteries get clogged, the greater the chances of suffering from a stroke or cardiac arrest. From this research, they concluded that cholesterol was to blame for heart problems because the arteries were clogged by that. This is why it was told to people that if they ate cholesterol-rich foods it would increase their body levels and thus cause heart ailments. Naturally, people began to demonize the red meat, butter, eggs and other foods high in cholesterol.

Nonetheless, do high cholesterol foods affect body levels? The answer is no since your body already knows how to control cholesterol levels. Because cholesterol is produced by the human body itself, it has its mechanism for maintaining a healthy body level. This acts like a feedback mechanism where the body avoids processing cholesterol when it becomes conscious that there are already high levels of it. Likewise, if cholesterol levels go down, the body will produce more of it.

What you must realize is that not all cholesterol is evil. There is good cholesterol as well as bad cholesterol. You need to pay attention to that. Cholesterol occurs as a molecule of fat and it is not soluble like salt or sugar. This is why traveling through the body requires a medium since it will not dissolve in the blood itself. The lipoproteins are this channel used for cholesterol molecules. We are a mixed group of molecules, containing both protein and fat. When necessary, the principal function of lipoproteins is to transport cholesterol to organs or cells. There is a classification of two types among lipoproteins which are responsible for this transport of cholesterol. One is lipoprotein or HDL of high density, and the other, lipoprotein or LDL of low density. Although it is not theoretically possible to call the HDL and LDL cholesterol, they are known as good and bad cholesterol.

HDL molecules have the function of transporting cholesterol from various parts of your body into your liver. It is either absorbed in the liver, or reused for the body. The LDL molecules carry cholesterol from the liver towards the rest of the body. If your body has a high level of HDL or good cholesterol you are at lower risk for cardiovascular disease. Your diet should be rich in natural dietary fibers to boost HDL levels. This is why there is a positive effect of a low carbohydrate diet by increasing HDL levels.

On the other hand, the LDL level shouldn't be high, and that's why it's called bad cholesterol, but it's just a low-density lipoprotein and not cholesterol really. The LDL itself is responsible for the conveyance of cholesterol, and when this level is high, more cholesterol is taken to the liver. Higher levels of LDL are responsible for the increased risk of heart ailments. Additionally the smaller LDL particles contribute to this negative impact. When you eat a low carb diet, it helps transform these into larger molecules and also leads to a reduction of LDL in your blood. By now you can understand that a healthy diet that is high in fat does not cause cholesterol problems. That type of diet allows for a healthier amount of cholesterol in the body.

We are also cautious of triglyceride levels, as it is cholesterol. But most of the triglyceride-related concerns are relatively unfounded. Triglycerides are a type of fat found most in food. They help to supply body oxygen. The only difference is that they will be used for future use as fuel storage and not for immediate body use.

As the body breaks down carbohydrates for energy use, some of these are processed as triglycerides in cells. The more carbohydrates the body deals with, the greater the insulin it produces. Too much insulin will cause blood sugar problems in the body and this will then increase the levels of triglycerides stored. So, you do not need to think about the fats again. Eating a low carbohydrate diet will help prevent any such issues. For this reason, the carnivorous diet removes carbohydrates and helps maintain good health.

CHAPTER 4: CHOOSING THE CARNIVORE DIET

I had no trouble in transitioning to a Carnivore Diet. It was in fact one of the easiest things I've ever done. It felt like I was moving into something that was more normal. I was excited to try it too, so my motivation was fueled by the excitement. I loved the food, I felt satisfied, I felt great despite a bit of "keto-flu" (see below I would say that I hear both sides when it comes to the ease or difficulty of transitioning to a Carnivore Diet. Many say it was easy mostly because they love beef, cheese, and bacon so much. Others have a hard time the first 3 to 10 days. The body is experiencing changes as it adapts to fat burning and it's not always enjoyable. During that first week (or two, or three!), you should anticipate changes in appetite, energy and focus levels. Eventually things should get back to normal.

My own keto-flu experience, coming from a "healthy" diet in Real-Food, was pretty minimal. The first 3 days I was more drained. I also had a headache, but I can't tell for sure if it was due to a change in eating versus a sinus headache caused by something different.

There are things that can help reduce the effects of keto-flu or make them less apparent. Here are some options:

Ease Into It Slowly

One way of gradually reducing the severity of keto-flu symptoms, as well as mental adjustment, is simply to gradually ease it in. Start by making all the break-fasts carnivore, instead of going cold-turkey. Allow carnivore after a week of all the breakfasts and lunches. Wait another week and do all the carnivore breakfasts, lunches and dinners.

This is just a sample; there are obviously other timetables and ways to slowly ease into it. Only feel free to become imaginative. Another way could be to start cutting out the refined carbs first from all meals. Swap grains with fruits and vegetables, then move toward all meat, etc.

Start on a weekend or holiday

You might prefer to start a Carnivore Diet during a time when you don't have to work or have severe commitments for other things. This could mean a long weekend away from work, or better yet, on the weekend. That way it is easier to tolerate if there are keto-flu symptoms.

On the other hand, it may be that certain people prefer job disruptions.

Allow More Time for Sleep

While I found myself in need of less sleep immediately, even from the first night, it's prudent to allow at least the extra rest. Over the first few days of change a nap may be in order.

Have the Right Expectations

If this is a dramatic change then through the transition period it could be both radically fantastic and bad at the same time. The grandeur of weight loss, mixed with the crappiness of being exhausted or getting headaches.

Expectations with the Carnivore Diet are not stopped though. If you're on the Carnivore Diet and you're living with your family or friends, it's also a good idea to help them have the right expectations.

My favorite approach to this is telling others I'm trying something new to feel better and to give me support please. Sometimes just asking for support is all a person needs to disarm the deniers. It's helpful to understand where these people come from too. If people don't support the diet, it's generally based on fear (which in most situations is just ignorance), or envy. If it is based on ignorance, you might be able to present useful information as to why the Carnivore Diet might be a good choice. If it's based on envy, well, it is a strategy perhaps to persuade the individual to do it together.

Anyway, I find that just asking for support straight up is a great way for people to be on the side of the Carnivore Diet.

Stay Hydrated

Not only is this necessary, but it is a good hack during cravings. I keep a large jug of water on my counter and my goal is to finish it by the end of the day (not to drink too far into the evening, or I'll have to pee in the middle of the night). This water is the first thing I see when I go into the kitchen, which reminds me to be drinking. Staying hydrated this way helps me drink less coffee, keep satiated and feel good.

Keep a Food Journal

I found it was helpful in the transition phase to log my daily food intake and experiences.

Journaling made me feel inspired. It also helped me to keep track of it all and make adjustments as needed.

Eat a Flex-Meal or Have a Flex-Day

A flex-meal or flex-day simply means allowing yourself a meal or day to eat whatever you want when you go off the Carnivore Diet. For example, you could do it once a week.

This option is to add stress-free flexibility. If the occasion arises you have allowances for some plants. Nevertheless, I do not recommend doing a flex-anything if it tends to start a cascade of carbohydrate cravings, as some people can have had happen.

HOW Does THE CARNIVORE DIET STARTS?

If you want to try the Carnivore Diet for yourself, you've got to understand that you're not going to get immediate results. Every healthy diet demands that you step in and show results for at least a few weeks. You may start the

Carnivore Diet with a one month target. If you see it working, and notice no bad side effects, you can go on from there. Take notes on how you feel in terms of things like strength, hunger cravings, etc. in the month, and also mark your weight down every week. You should take advantage of this opportunity to be curious about the diet and see how it works. A health diary is a great way of marking progress and keeping motivated. In this segment we'll try to help you continue the Carnivore Diet.

Carnivore Diet Stages

The Carnivore Diet can be divided into three stages, and this segment will help you get to know them. You can opt to do one stage at a time when you start the Carnivore Diet, or just start from the second stage if it suits you better. We'll help you understand what's involved in each stage, and more.

Stage One

You can eat any kind of meat or seafood you wish at this stage. Tea or coffee isn't restricted. You can eat cheese, butter, eggs or even heavy cream. This is the stage that allows the body to adjust to the Carnivore Diet and allows you to add additional supplements to help you in the process. Electrolytes are also advised to combat the diuretic effect of the Carnivore Diet on the body; however, it should be kosher even if you are using salt. The kosher salt law is valid during any point of the diet.

Stage Two

With two exceptions, anything that you do in stage one is allowed on stage two. At this point in the diet, you have to rule out all processed meats. It includes all the bacon, sausages, cold cuts, salami, etc. You also need to stop drinking coffee and tea as there was enough time to get rid of the habit during the adaptation period; however, this second aspect is not as important as giving up processed meat which is not safe for you.

Stage Three

It's a little tougher for you at this stage in the process, but if you want the Carnivore Diet to function for you optimally it needs to be worked through. Eliminate all foods and beverages, except beef and water, in your diet. Much research has shown that whilst following this diet, beef is the healthiest option. Since we've already removed processed meat, you need to find a place where organic grass-fed meat is sold. At this point give up any meat or seafood other than beef; however, if it is too costly, don't emphasize the grass-fed source. Seek just to stick to eating just watered beef. There are different cuts of beef that you can keep switching so you don't get bored with the diet.

In the first 30 days of starting the Carnivore Diet follow these three stages. At this point, don't try to tinker with the diet so you can adapt well and it works optimally for you. You're able to customize it after the 30 days to suit your lifestyle and needs. Experiment with permitted foods, and see what works best for you. You will notice that some types of food even within the diet will help you lose weight, while others may make you gain a little. So if you are trying to maintain a healthier body, limit your intake accordingly.

Do it step by step, when you start customizing after stage three. Start with adding fresh beef to your diet of grass-fed beef. Then also begin adding other animal meat or seafood; however, go with one meat added at a time. Following this you can begin to incorporate eggs into your diet, followed by other approved dairy products. Check what works and what doesn't work for you. In the end, if you managed to cut the habit by stage two, you can also start drinking a little tea or coffee too.

It gives you time to consider how your body reacts to a particular food when you are adding a single food at a time. If you see any unfavorable effect, try restricting or limiting its consumption. This is why many people are omitting pork when they see that it is causing a bit of weight gain. If there are any other ill effects like food allergies, you may also omit a food. You may find bloating when it comes to certain dairy products. In this situation, the food that causes bloating in your body should be eliminated; but, when it comes to eggs, we recommend adding them into your diet. Other than all of this, go ahead and tailor your diet plan according to your objectives. Be careful, and go one at a time through all of the stages.

On a more general note, follow the points set out below as a reference along with following stages described above.

What to eat first off, you need to find out everything on this diet you're allowed to eat. Anything that is not on the Carnivore's Diet list should not be consumed for at least the one month you set your goal for. As you already know, you are only allowed to eat meat from animals primarily. It's a diet of 100 per cent meat meals. There is no space for plant-based foods, or even protein product sources such as soy protein. As you'll know later in the book, certain dairy products are sometimes allowed, but if you choose, even this can be omitted.

Once you stock up on your meat-centric food list, get rid of all the processed food from your kitchen or workshop. There shouldn't be plant-sourced food either, so you can give your food to your friends or even to the nearby homeless shelter. Note that sugar, sauces, and other condiments should not be included in your diet either. Unless someone else in your house consumes all of this, get it out of sight. This will not encourage you not to fall into your old habits.

How much to eat

After you're certain of the foods permitted on the Carnivore Diet, you can stock up on them and start. You may be worried at this point about how much you are allowed to eat, or not. Well, the great thing about this diet is that there's no restriction on how much food there is. You shouldn't overeat, of course, but you can eat until you feel satiated. You don't want to be starving just because you think it's going to help you lose weight. Eat when you're hungry, because it's the way the body tells you that it needs more strength and calories. As you start the meat diet, you'll learn to differentiate real hunger from psychological hunger.

You'll see improvements in your appetite pattern over this first month. Your cravings and untimely appetite will be reduced and replaced by a more appropriate eating habit. This will also help you eat less and burn fat, too. You can assess how much food you need in a day by how much activity you do. Have enough meat to keep you going through the day if you have a more sedentary life, but avoid eating too much.

If you are a very active person or engage in daily sports, you may even need twice as much food as the average person. Accordingly you can decide how much food you need for yourself. You can eat less on certain days than on another day because you eat more because you've been very busy all day. You just need to remember and eat when you're hungry and eat until you're satisfied. Try not to eat less, and remain hungry. Instead, eat your fill and avoid eating in between meals. Don't try to over-stuff yourself either, learn to listen to your body. This will help you understand when you need food. You should usually eat 2-4 lbs. of meat in a day.

When to Eat

The next thing to remember is what time to eat or when to eat. Ideally three main meals are more than enough in the day. You should also try to set a schedule so you eat each day at the same time, as this will further benefit your health. The timing of each individual will depend on his / her daily schedule. Try to ensure you're eating a healthy morning protein-based breakfast to maintain your energy levels throughout the day. Set aside time to eat your lunch, no matter how busy you are in the work.

Take your own car, so you can avoid breaking your diet restrictions. Practice conscientious cooking, as well, and don't try multitasking and working while eating lunch. You may have dinner a few hours before you go to bed, once you're finished. When you feel hungry amongst any meal, try drinking water and eat a little more food if you are still hungry. But remember to always stick with foods approved for the diet.

What to drink

Preferably, if you are on a Carnivore Diet you should only drink water. Avoid drinking any other liquid for this first month of trial at least. Do not buy any branded beverages that say either low fat, no sugar or health drink. This can only be tap water, spring water, mineral water or even filtered water, but nothing with any flavoring or sugars. If you are unable to give up on your regular coffee or tea dose, make sure you don't add any sugar or artificial sweeteners. For the second and third stage of the diet, you should give these up, but some people continue afterwards. Sodas, juices, protein shakes, etc., are off limits in this diet. Whatever diet you are on, water is always the best way to stay hydrated. This helps to lose weight quicker, and prevents water retention from bloating.

How to Cook

There is typically no clear rule on how you cook. If you like your steak rare, eat it that way, but if you'd rather have it cooked well, that works too. Whatever meat or fish you cook, just make sure it's done in such a way that the food is safe to eat. When left uncooked and eaten, some forms of meat can make you ill. On the other side, there are a few forms which can also be eaten raw. For starters, if you like, you can eat raw salmon sushi, or fresh oysters. Also, as you eat meat most of the time, invest in some good meat cutting knives and a board intended for that purpose. Vegetable knives are quite hard to use when you want to slice certain kinds of tough cuts.

Common mistakes

A lot of people who want to lose weight often eat too little even when the diet doesn't restrict the amount of food they eat. Starving yourself won't make you lose weight healthily and will cause illness instead. Drink enough to satiate your thirst, and you'll find the diet itself helps to normalize your appetite over time. You must also remember, to stay hydrated all day long. This is intended to prevent fatigue and to aid in healthy body functions. Don't cut off salt from your diet completely, as this may cause symptoms of Keto flu that some people experience. Also, don't try to alter your own diet and add fruit or vegetables just because you were told they were healthy. If you want to see real Carnivore Diet results, you need to make sure you follow it properly. Another common mistake is avoiding fatty meat due to cholesterol reasons. Fatty meat is recommended for this diet and will deliver good cholesterol to your body. The diet will work well for you as long as you avoid certain kinds of mistakes.

FIND SUPPORT

If you find this diet or any diet difficult to follow, or if you are going through it, get help. Don't just try to get past it alone. Everyone knows how difficult it can be to break every habit or create new ones. In fact, the weight-loss process can be a very challenging one. In such moments, find a source of help such as family or friends with whom you are at ease. If not, then there are a lot of online support groups that can benefit you. Do whatever it takes to stay happy and healthy. Most Carnivore Dieting sites can help you meet other people like you, who can help you out.

Deciding on a long-term or short-term diet

You will wonder if the diet is healthy to adopt for the long-term. The Carnivore Diet is usually used by people on a short-term basis to help them lose weight; but, if you look at online forums and testimonials, you can find that many people have been practicing the diet for years and have enjoyed a healthy life. There are always exceptions to the rule, and there may be a problem with certain health conditions, so consult your doctor to find out if you can safely follow this meat-centered diet for longer than you originally intended.

Carnivore Diet Optimization

Every diet can be tailored for a person and for their intended purpose. If you want to lose weight while getting healthy, the following tips will help you optimize the diet for yourself.

Eat eggs

Try to add eggs to your diet even if it's an all meat diet. Eggs are permitted and we would recommend them. They contain a lot of nutrients which your body will benefit from. So cook eggs in different ways, and try to add them once in a while to your diet.

Eat offal

Many people usually overlook offal and avoid its consumption, but trust us when we say it is good for your health. Offal like the liver is extremely rich in vital nutrients like folate, Vitamin A, choline and iron. Eating a liver from animals is like taking a natural multivitamin for your body. Additionally, you should eat fish liver, which is both a healthy source of Vitamin D and B12.

More fish

Don't eat only red meat. The all-meat diet requires fish and supports its safe consumption. Seafood is a nutrient-rich supplement to a carnivorous diet. These contain a lot of fatty acids such as omega 3, iron, copper, manganese and Vitamin D. Seafood is an uncommon source of selenium that is deficient in most people's diets, but is needed for good health. The omega 3s extracted from fish will help your heart health in particular.

There are no restrictions on what seafood you should or shouldn't eat, so make them a regular part of your diet; however, just like meat, you should buy freshly caught fish from the wild and not those from fish farms. The latter is more likely to have been fed with chemicals or hormones to grow faster, and these will get into your diet too. We do understand that some people before did not have fish as part of their diet, so we suggest that you try it for a while by eating different varieties and using different cooking styles. Various fish oil supplements should work well for those who do choose not to eat the fish. Your ultimate goal is to eat as many nutrients as you can to optimize your health while following a Carnivore Diet.

Intermittent fasting

This is explained in detail in another section of the book. We highly recommend that you try and see the best results along with the Carnivore Diet. Fasting isn't the same as a diet of starvation, and it will benefit you in different ways. This technique and the Carnivore Diet will make more changes in the body. The output of your growth hormone will increase while both blood sugar and insulin will decrease. People generally choose to add intermittent fasting to their routine, since it is ideal to quickening the weight loss process. It will help your metabolic system and will have an enhanced effect on the immune system. Read the Intermittent Fasting section to read in depth about it.

Zero-calorie plant foods

Spices are a type of plant-sourced foods not containing calories. Therefore, they are in the grey area when it comes to plant foods. These can be used along with herbs to improve the flavor of your meat-based diet. The herbs and spices have an added nutritional value to your diet. We even use a variety of herbs such as rosemary as herbal supplements.

Good meat quality

Even with a meat based diet, quality matters. Eating just any meat product at random won't be ideal for your health. Sourcing meat of the best quality will help with your intent. Grass-fed meat or pastured meat is far better than any factory-farmed meat. The latter are fed hormones that accumulate in your body, or chemicals that harm you in the long run. The same principle applies to seafood, which should be caught fresh and not bought from farm fishing.

Bone Broth

As we mentioned earlier, bone broth is one of the liquids other than water permitted among liquids. Adding bone broth to your diet will bring many different benefits. It is an excellent source of collagen, which is important for healthy skin and bone.

Get your blood tested before you start following a Carnivore Diet.

Repeat after a couple of weeks of following the diet. It will help you gage the impact it has on your body. You need to take note of weight, energy level adjustments and even the digestive functions. The first week of adaptation may be a little tough, because your strength and appetite fluctuate a lot and you may find it difficult to focus as well. Try to take a week off work, or start a week when there is less workload.

How to Stay On Track on the Carnivore Diet

Here are some tips that will help you stay on track when following your Carnivore Diet. We know how hard it can be to put food restrictions into your normal lifestyle all of a sudden. That's why staying on track can be too much for some people and they end up failing to reach their goals. At some point you might feel like quitting, or just losing focus. Therefore, the following approaches will assist you on your journey.

Visualization

This mental technique can be very successful. If you want to see some positive changes happening within yourself and your life, visualize it. You have to imagine kicking off your unhealthy dietary habits and successfully starting the Carnivore Diet. Picture how you want to look, and how you want to feel in a year or so. This image should help you stay motivated until you succeed in getting it done. You can even imagine yourself in a dress that right now doesn't fit you, but looks stunning on you in the near future.

Be realistic

You should always have achievable and realistic expectations. You set yourself up to disappointment and failure when you set unrealistic expectations. If you want to lose weight, find a healthy target every month. A few pounds in a month is a safe, achievable target. But if you think in a couple of months you'll lose 10 pounds, that's probably unrealistic. Manageable goals are easier and safer to achieve.

CHAPTER 5: USING THE CARNIVORE DIET TO LOSE WEIGHT, INTERMITTENT FASTING METHOD

If you want to lose weight after starting the Carnivore Diet, then you should also try to implement intermittent fasting into your routine. Fasting is a ritual that has been practiced in various cultures around the world since ancient times. Nonetheless, do not confuse fasting with starving. Intermittent fasting doesn't work like a fad diet which tells you to starve to lose five pounds in a week. The latter is a completely unreasonable practice which will affect your health negatively. On the other hand, intermittent fasting is beneficial to your health and is a recommended addition to your diet to just help in the weight loss process.

Intermittent fasting is an effective way to make the Carnivore Diet more effective in terms of both weight and health benefits. The protocol is quite clear, but it is true that it cannot be followed by everyone. But the benefits are likely to prompt you to at least try; however, we think you should only do this after the first month or so of starting the Carnivore Diet. The initial stage is already going to be a drastic change you need to adapt to. In this initial phase, if you try to tinker with the diet, it will get much harder for you. So try intermittent fasting once that process is over.

Next, you need to find out what intermittent fasting is. It is a technique where you follow a diet with intermittent periods in which no eating is permitted. These could be a no-food period of anything in a day, between 15 and 24 hours. But at one time you're allowed to fast over a day. This is how a starvation diet or some unhealthy fad diet is different. You're only taught how to prevent yourself from eating and observe a fast time every couple of days in a week. It may sound tough right now, particularly if you've never fasted before, but it isn't. Many people have tried intermittent fasting in order to lose weight and for its different health benefits. They've found it effective, and we recommend it to help you more effectively along with the Carnivore Diet. You will be able to lose weight much faster, improve your metabolism, muscle gain and maintain a healthy weight afterwards.

Intermittent fasting is a flexible plan, adaptable to one's health and needs. It can vary from person to person so that according to your ability you can implement a plan for the fast. While the Carnivore Diet concentrates more on what you consume, intermittent fasting lets you control how much food you eat. This way you exercise control over both the quality and the amount of food.

Most of us have an unhealthy habit of eating and overeating at the wrong time by skipping meals in time. In this respect, the intermittent fasting plan helps us exercise more discipline. It can be of great help to those who have a poor habit of giving in to cravings or over-consumption. You will automatically eat less when you have restricted eating periods on your diet, so you'll see results faster than just following the Carnivore Diet alone.

You can choose a different method of intermittent fasting, depending on the type of lifestyle you lead. Having a diet that suits you personally will help you carry it through. Many people don't realize how important it is to heed their individual needs. You can't expect the same plan to work for you that worked for someone else. That's why there are different types of intermittent fasting from which we let you pick. In fact, you are even allowed to eat in some of these, albeit in limited quantities.

LEAN GAIN METHOD

The lean gain diet is one method of intermittent fasting. In this type you are allowed to eat for 8 hours a day, while the rest of the 16 hours must be a period of fasting. There's no timing specification provided in the day, so you can change this according to your schedule. In the fasting period, all you need to make sure there is no food. You can also change the diet accordingly. If you do a lot of exercise on a given day, you can add more fat to a meal. Look for more protein and reduce the fat on a more sedentary day. This helps keep your balance healthy.

WEEKLY METHOD

You just have to fast for one day in the week in this type of intermittent fasting. In a seven-day week, that means a 24-hour fast. The remainder of the 6 days will be the normal diet plan for carnivores. Again there are no specified timings. If you want to, you can start in the morning, or even after lunch. Just ensure from that time onwards there is a 24-hour fast. This is one of the easier types to follow and even the beginners can try it out. This one-day fast serves as a boost to improve your healthy diet.

ALTERNATE DAY METHOD

This is another type of intermittent fasting, but it does not require you to omit food completely at any point. Alternatively, one day you are supposed to eat regularly while the next day should require limited eating. This cycle will continue as every Minimum Eating alternative day. You should be concentrating on eating half of what you usually eat over these days. You shouldn't focus on filling your stomach as you usually do, and just eat a little more. Don't try to overeat the next day to make up for less food on your fasting day.

WARRIOR METHOD

Simple and quite common warrior method. You have to fast for about 20 hours a day in this kind of intermittent fasting, with 4 hours free to eat as you please. Don't be offset by the idea of the 20-hour fasting period, as the warrior method allows you to eat a little even in those hours, but very minimally. It is also recommended that you eat more at night, rather than during the day.

If you find all these kinds of fasts difficult, just try to practice a little fasting every now and then. On the first day, you can begin by placing a restriction on food for a duration of 15 hours. Start the morning with your fast, and have a meal and sleep when you break your fast. This way you're not going to go to sleep hungry, and that's going to be easier for you. If it is tough for you, you can do this once a week. Following two days of regular eating you can then try it again. In a week later, that way, you will try for three days of intermittent fasting; however, make sure that you do not fast consistently for two days at a time or more than 3-4 days a week.

You might find it difficult the first few days you try intermittent fasting. There is a period of adaptation which will take a few days. Give yourself an opportunity to get through this initial phase and you'll find it much easier. Be soft on yourself, and do not immediately attempt to impose strict restrictions. Your body is already undergoing a transition with the Carnivore Diet so it will induce unnecessary stress. Remember, don't consider using this as an excuse to starve yourself because you think it's going to help you get thin faster. Not providing adequate food for your body will just harm you. Then adopt your Carnivore Diet with a balanced schedule of intermittent fasting once in a while.

HELPFUL NOTES IN INTERMITTENT FASTING:

Eat enough of the foods allowed on the Carnivore Diet when it is not a day of fasting. Don't over-eat to make up for fasting, but don't eat too much either. If you practice fasting it will just make it harder for you.

Try drinking some green tea if you feel hungry during a no-food period. That will help to curb the pangs of hunger. Do not add sweetener to this. Drinking black coffee will boost your body too.

Try to stay hydrated, whether it is a day of fasting or not. In particular, dehydration on a fasting day can be very damaging to your health. Always have a little water at hand. You can even add some electrolytes if you feel nauseous or faint.

Eat healthy sources of dietary fat as recommended in carnivorous diets. Butter or eggs aren't your enemy and will do you good.

Benefits of intermittent fasting:

Weight loss

Generally, help in weight loss is the main goal behind attempting intermittent fasting. Thankfully it fulfills the intent and is not in any way a waste of effort. This decreases your food intake, which in turn means you consume less calories; but, if you try to make up for a fasting day by overeating on the other days, this won't hold true. It also improves hormone functioning which promotes weight loss. Since insulin levels are lowering with an increase in nor-adrenaline and growth hormone, fat molecules are further breaking down. Calorie intake is reduced when maximizing metabolic activity. One of the best parts is that it helps in particular to lose weight from the belly, which could otherwise be difficult.

Increased insulin resistance

Intermittent Carnivore Diet fasting can help people who are at risk of or suffer from type 2 diabetes. If a person has type 2 diabetes their level of blood sugar is high and their body's resistance to insulin increases. This can be very harmful to health and cause additional illnesses. Intermittent fasting has been known to help lower blood sugar levels as well as to reduce insulin resistance.

Increased inflammation

If your body has a lot of oxidative stress, it will increase the aging rate and also increase the risk of multiple chronic conditions. The oxidative stress is caused by unstable molecules that interfere with stable protein or DNA molecules. This then destroys the molecules that are healthy and hurts the body. Including intermittent fasting will help improve your body's resistance to conditions like these.

Improved heart condition

Over the last few decades heart disease has risen alarmingly. One of the main causes of that is a bad diet. High blood pressure, bad cholesterol, high triglyceride levels and high blood sugar increase the risk of heart disease;

intermittent fasting, however, helps to reduce the risk associated with all of these and thus improves heart health.

Cell function

Food plays a lot of different roles in your body. If you don't eat enough during a given period, the cells in the body will be prompted to start repairing or regenerating. Your body's hormonal levels will change, and they'll work to also make your body burn fat for energy. The drop-in insulin level also makes this burning fat process easier. Alternatively, growth hormone will rise in the body too. A positive change will be seen in the composition of genes and molecules which sustain a long healthy life. This will strengthen the immune system, as well. Often cells begin removing waste during the fasting cycle. Dysfunctional cells and proteins are broken down in the course of an autophagy process. The risk of diseases such as cancer and Alzheimer's has been known to decrease as autophagy increases. This promotes the removal of waste build-up in cells.

To some people, incorporating more meat-based meals gradually over time is a good transition strategy. Another example of this is the distribution of three meat-based meals throughout the first week. Up to eight carnivore meals bump up to next week. Seek only meat based meals for two days in the third week, and spread 10 carnivore meals on the other days. You should be able to handle five days of carnivore meals within the fourth week, and by the fifth week, all but two of your meals will be meat.

Your transition to full carnivore will be complete within week six. Alternatively, three days out of a week, you could set short-term challenges in going full carnivore. The next challenge is to go one full week eating meat only. The third challenge is to go for two weeks; at last, for thirty days in a row, you are going to go carnivore. This method is something I used and it was a fairly smooth process.

The third gradual transition technique is to fade the vegetables and starch off your plate as you increase the amount of meat you eat every day.

One downside to these incremental approaches is that you still have exposure to addictive or otherwise unhealthy foods for some time, which can make it more difficult for you to let go of those things. It's kind of like drinking alcohol after just having alcohol twice a week. But, as long as you continue to move closer to a completely carnivorous diet, you'll probably feel better, and over time those cravings will subside.

The gradual withdrawal of fiber-or oxalate-rich foods could also promote the process. Through -removing fiber from your diet slowly, your colon can better adapt to be able to efficiently absorb fluids and minerals. Gradually tapering from oxalate-rich foods will help you avoid possible rapid oxalate crystal precipitation into your joints, skin or other tissues.

THE BEGINNER PHASE

How long will the starting phase last? It can differ, but here are some indications that classify a beginner from a seasoned carnivore:

• Food no longer controls you, and you no longer see food as a form of entertainment. It is a deeply satisfying source of nutrition, instead.

• You have no problem passing on a food which was one of your favorites before.

• You can go out socially and not press for something to eat just to appease somebody else.

• Nothing else would seem like food but meat.

Those signs are evident to some people within a few months. It takes years for other people to reach all of these milestones.

May I Change the Diet?

Any diet has many ways to tinker it. Purist proponents oppose any diet that deviates from the program, but some individuals will always make adjustments.

Many people can go about eating satiety for years (maybe even decades or a lifetime) and living on primarily fatty cuts of meat while being as happy and healthy as possible. Some people may break from the Carnivore Diet only to find out they need to stay aligned with the diet to prevent a relapse into bad habits or to prevent devastating health problems from returning. Most people who try this diet probably won't stay strictly carnivorous. Many will drift back and forth between the carnivorous diet and a more normal diet; they may even float around carnivorous or near carnivorous for much of their lives as they know that they are getting the best health and performance benefits the closer they are to being exclusively carnivorous, but they won't be 100 percent carnivores 100 percent of their time.

Like veganism advocates, who often have ethical reasons to adopt an all-plant diet, people following the Carnivore Diet do so for health and performance reasons. People on this diet don't try to save broccoli from extinction, or think they're making the world a better place. It's not a religion or a cult; it's simply a way to strive to be safe and get the best nutrition possible. Many people use the Carnivore Diet to solve health problems and fix problems — especially with their gut function— so that they can gradually return other to foods with no ill effect to their diets.

Other people use a strict carnivorous diet as an occasional tool, and some others may find that they feel optimal if they are "mostly carnivorous." I don't generally recommend that you tinker with the carnivorous diet until you have conquered all the demons that would keep you in the beginner phase. I suggest everyone spend at least a couple of months fully carnivorous before playing around with other things.

METABOLISM AND CALORIES

Do calories matter? Indeed, they do. If you ingest more calories than you burn, you lose mass. So how do you control the amount of calories you burn? What also affects your appetite, and how many calories do you ingest?

This question is the subject of much debate on both sides of the issue, with vocal advocates. Would you reduce your caloric intake actively, and increase your activity level? Absolutely, and an effective short-term strategy can be this. In the fitness community we see the facts all the time. Will some foods naturally satiate more than others? The answer is yes, and as demonstrated by the ever-increasing number of highly palatable, but ultimately unsatisfactory foods being manufactured and heavily marketed, the food industry is very aware of that fact. Can different people eat an identical number of calories and end up at different amounts of weight or lose differing amounts? Yes, of course, and even one person may see differences from one time to the next. Contrast a younger version of yourself, for example with the current version. Which one can eat more calories without weight gain? It was most probably your younger self.

Are we capable of shifting our metabolic efficiency? I think the answer is that we do, and I also believe that a carnivorous diet promotes some of that capacity. Carnivore Diet's effects on metabolism are likely due to improvements in insulin sensitivity, improvements in other hormones and improvements in cellular and mitochondrial functions. If a person transitioning to the Carnivore Diet is able to eat more food and maintain a healthy weight, equivalent to what that person might do when young, then he or she is likely to be metabolically normal.

A recent one-year Harvard study costing $12 million has shown that people could eat around 250 extra calories per day on a low-carbohydrate diet compared to a higher carbohydrate diet and not regain weight previously lost.

In fact, numerous studies indicate that as protein consumption rises, metabolic rates do so.

I often see people following the Carnivore Diet saying they eat a lot more calories in meat than they did in total before, but still lose weight.

I have no doubt this could happen; it possibly has to do with changes in some of the inefficiencies of the body. Protein is also particularly difficult to metabolically convert to fat. Diet, exercise, infrequent eating, and other methods can improve mitochondrial density. Ultimately having more mitochondria means better performance and better metabolic health. If you are hell-bent on getting to a very low level of body fat then it may be helpful to combine cycling macronutrients with a slight decrease in calories or an increase in activity.

A strong appetite is a good sign of health, especially when it doesn't lead to body fat gains. Once a person reaches this level of metabolic normalcy, then I think we see more alignment with what we see in the athletic and fitness community, with a more predictable response to compositions of macronutrients and caloric intake.

SPONTANEOUS USE OF THE CARNIVORE DIET

For some people— especially those who have no significant difficulties with food addictions, cravings or major health problems— cyclically following the Carnivore Diet may be a great option. This diet works well as a diet for removal. Those who have food allergies or gut health issues, and who turn to the Carnivore Diet are likely to have removed the food problem. After a person has been on a Carnivore Diet for some time, when those sensitivities have healed, the person can often begin eating other foods without experiencing any ill effects.

That's awesome if you're in this category of people; the carnivore police won't hunt you down and tell you to walk away from the blueberries or dark chocolate slice. You need to be frank with yourself though. Keep in mind that a healthy life needs none of the other foods. Your diet is focused on meat. If you choose to supplement your diet with another type of food, you should be very analytical about its effect.

I recommend you keep to single-ingredient foods as you reintroduce products into your diet. Try to eat one item and then wait several days to determine the impact of that meal. It may very well take three or more trials to get a clear sense of what's going on. Some adverse GI effects can simply reflect a gastrointestinal microbiome which is poorly prepared.

Let's say you've been a strict carnivore for six months, for example, and you've taken care of all of your health problems. At this point you would like to try to have some berries occasionally. I recommend you eat a small amount every day; write down any negative or positive outcomes from that experiment, critically. Wait 3 or 4 days, and repeat the process. Compare outcomes of both attempts. You can play with the quantity, if you seem to tolerate the berries. You may find that a small amount is ok, but a larger amount is problematic.

In most cases, people who have long been strict carnivores are pretty good at evaluating dietary effects on their wellbeing, mood, skin, joint pain, digestion and so on. You should have a list of suitable and health-promoting (or at least health-neutral) foods after several weeks or months of trials with different foods which you can use as part of your diet on a daily or cyclical basis. If six months go by and you find yourself a little worse for wear, by going back to being a strict carnivore, you can reestablish a baseline.

Surprisingly, most people who deviate from a strict carnivorous diet tend to remain relatively close to the program because they realize how strong and nutritionally fulfilling it is. In other words, although the reverse is often true, it is highly unlikely that a committed carnivore would eventually end up as a vegan.

CARNIVORE DIET AND PREGNANCY

Can a woman have a regular carnivorous diet during pregnancy? The short reply is yes. There are countless examples of women who have done that in modern times and we know, of course, that women have been doing it for thousands of years. It is certainly sensible to let your obstetrician know about your diet so you can add any recommended supplements or other foods you need during your pregnancy. Breastfeeding generally seems to go well after the baby is born and lactation problems do not appear to be common. If you're in the midst of a pregnancy, a sudden change in diet can be upsetting. I recommend that you make a gradual change if you plan to go down the route to the Carnivore Diet.

Kids can also use the Carnivore Diet. Sure, they would have adopted the eating style traditionally. Children have no nutritional requirements other than the adults. To put it another way, children need the same essential things we do.

Children can start their Carnivore Diet as soon as they are ready to wean away from breast milk. They can start with teething on bones and eating fine-cut or pureed meats. You need to be vigilant, of course, and use caution to ensure that no shock occurs.

It's often hard to control the kids' diet when they communicate with their peers, and frankly kids should have a choice about what they're eating;

they'll ultimately make their own decisions anyway. It helps to educate them about the benefits and potential problems with food choices very early on. My children sometimes choose to be completely carnivorous and I certainly do not discourage this practice. I'm making sure they always have access to plenty of well-prepared meat dishes that they give priority to over other foods.

If they want to eat something else, like fruit, vegetables or other similar whole foods, I don't discourage them after they have eaten their meat. I limit or try not to expose them to processed foods, sugars, vegetable oils and refined grain products. I typically send them off with full stomachs when they go to birthday parties or other "junk food" activities to eliminate the risk of eating a bunch of garbage. Other families have children that remain completely carnivorous, and the children seem to be doing well.

How do carnivorous athletes perform on a diet? Once, it seems the conclusion is they are thriving. World-class athlete Owen Franks, who played for the All Blacks rugby team in New Zealand, has followed a carnivorous diet, for example. He's seen his performance level boost and noticed higher strength levels and lean body mass. My athletic performance has improved very greatly, and since I have been completely carnivorous I have been able to set three world records in indoor rowing masters and six American records.

Numerous high-level athletes, including Olympic athletes, have approached me from a wide range of sports including weightlifting, powerlifting, mixed martial arts, jiu-jitsu, CrossFit, cycling, marathon running, cricket, rowing, shot put and rugby. All the athletes who have moved to the Carnivore Diet have recorded significant improvements in overall performance, better rehabilitation and quick injury healing. That said, some athletes notice a drop in performance during the transition period, which is often related to undereating or due to a need to adjust to the diet. This period can last for several weeks to several months; the length is somewhat dependent on the athlete's prior nutritional plan and the sport.

For example, a person who comes from a high-carbohydrate diet engaged in a highly glycolytically challenging sport like CrossFit or cycling may take longer to adapt than other athletes do. A person who has previously been on a ketogenic diet and is competing in powerlifting could have an easier transition.

ADVANTAGE / DISADVANTAGE OF THE CARNIVORE DIET

We'll take a look at some of the pros and cons of adopting this diet in this part of the book. It has its own advantages and drawbacks just like everything else or any other diet.

Carnivore Diet Disadvantages

One disadvantage of an all-meat diet is that it can harm your health rather than improve it if you don't eat good-quality meat. The cheaper processed meat is usually filled with many preservatives, residues, and chemicals. These animals are fed foods which are of low quality and filled with toxins such as pesticides, GMOs, antibiotics, etc. that then enter their bodies. So you will also eat all of these indirectly from the low-quality meat. Therefore, it is important to find meat from animals grown in pastures, which are grass-fed or fed organic foods. This will ensure that the animals, and so their meat, are safe. If you follow a meat-based diet this factor is essential.

As meat contains a lot of saturated fat and cholesterol, you will regularly get a lot of that in your diet. That could be a disadvantage. This diet's trans-fat may also cause the liver to generate more cholesterol than it requires. This is why you have to control the amount of fatty meat you regularly consume.

Another drawback is the high sodium level found in processed meats or salted meats. Excessive sodium intake can increase the risk of heart disease or stroke, and can even be a kidney function problem. That's why it's recommended to avoid processed meat such as salami, jerky, or ham to avoid excess sodium. Fresh meat will have much lower sodium levels, and is not a problem.

When you look at the cost factor it is true that a meat diet is more costly than a diet based on plants. The diet can be quite costly if you're not only doing food for yourself, but for the whole family. Buying meat on a daily basis is expensive, especially if you want the kind of good quality. You should be prepared to increase expenditure on food in your budget unless you have your own farm animals or can process the meat yourself in any way. One tip that will help is to buy in bulk, as it usually lowers costs.

Carnivore Diet Advantages

This diet has the advantage that it is fairly simple. It saves you a lot of time and energy, since both your ingredients and the process of cooking are simplified. Not only will you see improvement in your health, but you will also notice that you spend a lot less of your day preparing food in the kitchen. If you adopt the Carnivore Diet, most of the cutting, grinding, and cooking parts that are involved in your normal day are omitted.

The Carnivore Diet is an important protein source for the body. Protein is essential to keep a lot of the food in the body and keep it healthy. That's why it's considered a vital building block. Since you'll just eat meat, your body has a constant source of good protein. Even a small amount of meat is densely packed with protein, and will compensate for a person's recommended daily allowance.

You'll also get all of the essential amino acids your body requires. There are nine amino acids which the body cannot make even if they are necessary for health. The proteins in meat contain amino acids and in fact they have all nine. That's why animal meat is considered a full source of protein and provides the body through the diet with these essential amino acids. Such amino acids need to be eaten frequently for the maintenance of healthy bones, muscle and skin.

A good source of B-complex vitamins like niacin, riboflavin, thiamine, and Vitamin B12 will also be obtained. All of these are contained in meat and thus help to maintain energy levels and contribute to growth. These vitamins also help absorb iron more effectively. Meat will also provide your body with other minerals, such as zinc and selenium.

Another benefit is that this diet has helped many people overcome certain chronic diseases which they would otherwise not be able to treat. This includes autoimmune diseases and Lyme disease. This diet helped a lot of people get healthier on a purely meat-based diet when other treatments and even a good doctor's protocol failed.

CHAPTER 6: COMPARISONS

DIFFERENCE BETWEEN KETO DIET, PALEO DIET AND CARNIVORE DIET

As you know, the Carnivore Diet is often compared to the low carb and keto diet, but at a certain point the overlap with similarities between those diets ends.

Firstly, let's look at what each of these diets entails.

The Paleo Diet

In a nutshell, this diet says you shouldn't eat any food a caveman didn't eat. When you decide to follow the Paleo Diet, you'll be allowed to eat anything that cave dwellers would hunt or collect and eat in their diet. That will include regional-growing meat, nuts, fish, seeds, leafy greens and vegetables. You're going to have to give up all the processed food that's part of the diet today. This means they have to give up pasta, candy, cereals, etc. This diet doesn't tell you how much you should eat and also doesn't set any limits on calories for the day. Rather, it's focused on improving the kind of food you eat.

Ketogenic Diet

The Keto Diet is basically low in carbs and high in fat and allows moderate protein intake. In fact, it is quite similar to other low carb diets, such as the Atkins diet. This diet has the intention of eating a lot of fat and putting your body in a constant state of ketosis. This ketosis process will push your body to burn up the stored fat in your body as a source of energy. Your body will turn to ketones, rather than glucose. Instead, the diet pushes your metabolic system away from its reliance on carbs towards ketones and fat. There are a few versions of the Keto Diet which can be adjusted in a day to suit the activity level of the person.

The Carnivore Diet

The Carnivore Diet is not about macros and focuses entirely on one food: meat. You're simply supposed to eat meat in this diet for all your meals, and no other foods. The only exception is a small amount of freshly processed dairy products.

When it comes to weight loss, most popular diets will tell you to eat fewer carbs. The Keto Diet decreases the carb intake while the Carnivore Diet eliminates carbohydrates from your diet entirely. How do you decide which one would be better? The Paleo Diet advocates plant-based foods, but does not contain gluten-like toxins and irritants. Does that mean the Carnivore Diet is the best meat-only choice then? There are groups of people who agree with this last synopsis and there are others who are totally opposed to it; however, you are probably in the middle since you can see that the

Carnivore Diet has its own unique advantages and can help you get lean and balanced.

The carbohydrate requirements of the Carnivore Diet are probably much more severe than you can see in a Keto Diet. The Keto Diet includes a modest amount of protein with a high fat content and a small amount of carbohydrates. In the case of Carnivore Diet, you will almost solely eat proteins and fats.

There was not a more extensive study on the Carnivore Diet compared with the Keto Diet. The Keto Diet has long been studied and therefore has a lot of scientific support; however, the same effort has not been put into understanding the Carnivore Diet. That's why there's no such reliable ratio to instruct you on how much fat and protein you can eat on your Carnivore Diet.

The Keto Diet, on the other hand, typically has a regular ratio to determine the amount of fats, proteins, and carbs that you need to eat every day. The normal ratio in a Keto Diet is 60-70 per cent fat, 20-30 per cent protein and 5-10 per cent carbohydrates. The Carnivore Diet lets you eat without any restrictions on macronutrients.

The only time carbs are allowed in the Carnivore Diet if they come in the form of fresh dairy products. There are certain fresh or fermented dairy products which contain a decent amount of carbs. While the Carnivore Diet requires this source of carbs, there are many who don't even eat that. You may have low carb vegetables in a Keto Diet but this is not permitted on the Carnivore Diet; however, we recommend that you follow a healthier approach that balances the amount of meat you eat with certain animal products such as eggs or milk. This will allow the Carnivore Diet to have a healthier approach.

The Paleo and Keto Diet allows a certain number of spices, salt, oils, etc. that help to add value as well as taste to your meals; however, it is slightly debatable in the Carnivore Diet whether or not these are allowed. These ingredients come from plants and the diet for carnivores emphasizes eating only animal-sourced food.

The Ketogenic Diet is a low carb diet whereas the Carnivore Diet completely eliminated carbohydrates. For this reason the latter is considered far more conservative than Keto. In the Keto Diet you can also eat plant foods which include nuts and seeds. Like Keto, the Carnivore Diet limits all of that. On the other hand, some high carb foods are restricted on the Keto Diet, but these are permitted on the Carnivore Diet so long as they are taken from an animal source. Since these dairy products are to be eaten minimally anyhow, the amount of carbs in the food is not of consequence.

People usually adopt the Carnivore Diet as a last resort as compared with the other two diets. Also, this diet is taken up when the other diets don't work or offer effective results. People who are suffering from health problems such as chronic pain or digestive problems often seek the Carnivore Diet to see if it will help to relieve those problems. After somebody's tried Paleo, Keto, intermittent fasting and many other diets, they're finally open to trying out a more extreme diet like this all meat one; however, like other diets, it's going to work for some people and not so much for others.

WHO SHOUD USE THE CARNIVORE DIET?

You might wonder if this meat-centered diet is right for you, or not. With some exceptions to the rule we recommend that you try it. You will find out more about who will benefit from this diet in this section, and who should not follow it. Until entering into the diet and removing all other items, you can consult a physician or dietician who will review your health and medical records to decide what's right for you. Everyone can have a plan that's optimized to suit their particular needs.

The Carnivore Diet is typically more commonly prescribed for those suffering from certain food intolerances. The diet is prescribed for such people on a short-term basis to help them discover what foods potentially aggravate their condition. You can slowly introduce new foods into your diet and keep checking which impacts your health negatively. Most people found the diet to be beneficial in that respect. A lot of people suffer from food intolerances, so they find the Carnivore Diet helpful in reducing the associated negative symptoms.

The aversion is a negative reaction that happens when the person consumes a particular food or even a certain food group. The wheat or dairy products cause some of the most common food intolerances. This will mean that in those foods like gluten or lactose, such people have intolerance to a substance. Thus, by eliminating those foods they can prevent the symptoms.

Certain additives which could cause a problem are lectin or phytic acid which is usually found in plant foods. These ingredients can cause digestion problems; however, they are not included in the Carnivore Diet so you can identify which food causes the problem, excluding the meat you are eating. Similarly, you will eliminate all potential food intolerances and then re-introduce it slowly, one at a time. You'll learn what to remove from the diet when you experience the reaction your body has to any meal.

If you have high blood pressure, you may want to really try the Carnivore Diet. We'll send you an old account of the facts that this diet helps maintain better blood pressure levels. As we have told you before, Greenland's Inuit people originally adopted a carnivorous diet in nature. They ate lots of meat and fish, and very little vegetables or fruits. Their diet was quite high in animal fat; however, a few of these families wanted to immigrate to Denmark at some stage around the late 1900s.

As they migrated, a more modern Danish diet was introduced which consisted of more plant-based foods and dairy products. Their daily intake of meat and of animal-sourced foods was greatly reduced. This found, when research was done, that this improvement in their diet actually raised their blood pressure by more than ten points compared to the previous. They followed the advice that, as they moved to Denmark, we are all still fed on a healthy diet; however, this showed that reducing meat did not actually help their blood pressure but increased it to an unhealthy level.

Research has shown that even among the Masai of Africa only 1 percent of men who adopted the meat diet suffered from high blood pressure. Throughout their lives, barely any of them had any problems, and blood pressure points only increased slightly when they crossed age 60. That's why we recommend you try to eat in the old Inuit or Masai tribe way to try and also improve your blood pressure levels.

The Carnivore Diet can also be of great benefit to those suffering from obesity or being overweight to an unhealthy extent. Obesity is a very modern-day disease indeed. When you look back in history, except among your own ancestors, there was hardly any mention of such overweight people. Modern-day diet is the main cause behind this weight-related disease, and the negative impact the food industry has had on it. Let's look to the Masai or Samburu people. There wasn't even obesity among those people when they followed the all-meat diet.

All these people had a suitable body weight, and it has been stable throughout their lives. You may say that you can see the Eskimos eating the all-meat diet and they look fat, but that's not true. In the peculiarity of their race, their features are healthy. It is not about being overweight or corpulent. They look a little healthier because of their puffy warm clothes which need to shield their bodies from the cold. Without these bulky clothes, when you see them, we assure you there are no unhealthy abdominal folds or bulging tummies. Such people are not immune to being obese but are safer because of the very lifestyle they are adopting.

If they moved to a city that had access to modern food, they would get overweight just as quickly as anyone else. You can see why we recommend the Carnivore Diet for people who are suffering from obesity, considering those instances. It may be difficult for obese people to follow other strict diets which require them to measure their portions or to regularly count their calories. We are often left frustrated and hungry by it.

Essentially, the diet is typically too difficult for most to follow through with; however, the Carnivore Diet makes it much simpler and easier to adopt long-term. The person is also allowed to eat as much as they need to satisfy their appetite, but it still helps lose a lot of the body's unhealthy fats. So at least try the Carnivore Diet for a few months, if you want to lose weight.

The Carnivore Diet also helps those with an increased risk of heart disease. As we mentioned in a previous chapter, a study on the people of Point Hope in Alaska proved this particular benefit of the diet. That region's people were largely untouched by the unhealthy modern diet, and continued to follow the meat or fish diet of the Eskimos. The study showed that the prevalence of cardiovascular problems was almost ten times lower compared with the population of the majority of the places in the US.

Who doesn't want to try it?

First of all, for people suffering from eating disorders, we do not recommend Carnivore Diet or any other strict diet. If you have had anorexia, bulimia or any of these conditions, work with a doctor to get a healthy diet that will help you recover. You have to prioritize your personal health and not your weight. You have to make more effort to instill positivity in your body. Go ahead, until the doctor says you're at a safe point and can follow the diet. But, without proper consultation, don't try.

The Carnivore Diet is also unfit for people suffering from any serious kidney disease. If you already have a serious kidney or other organ problem, your doctor will help you with the best diet possible. The diet can actually help improve functioning for those with a healthy kidney function as it helps get rid of excess glucose whilst improving insulin sensitivity.

Sportsmen and athletes may also wonder if they should follow the carnivorous diet. There is no appropriate research able to dictate this exactly. Many Carnivore Diet followers claim their strength improved on the diet. It does take the body time to get used to using meat for energy, though. The diet is not usually recommended for athletes because they continuously consume a high amount of energy. A low carb diet such as the Ketogenic diet can be modified to meet their needs, but the Carnivore Diet is much more stringent and may not be appropriate.

If you're curious if the diet is healthy to adopt, we'll respond in the affirmative, similar to any other diet under the same conditions. Many people react to certain diets better while others react differently. It has proved safe and effective for most of the people who have tried it. You do know that the main cause of increased heart disease is not animal fat but sugar, so you shouldn't think about this factor either; however, no long-term studies have been done on this diet, so you'll find no definitive evidence to prove it safe or unhealthy.

SIDE EFFECTS AND HOW TO DEAL WITH THEM

Following the ketogenic or Carnivore Diet means you can experience a side effect called Keto-flu. The Carnivore Diet will definitely benefit your health but your body needs time to get used to the change. You might have to contend with a variety of side effects, including Keto flu. We will explain everything in this part of the book about what it is, and how you can handle it.

In addition, Keto flu is a common side effect encountered during the initial phase of the Carnivore Diet. It is also known as induction flu and within the first week of the transition you can feel this. Nausea, lethargy, fatigue and lack of concentration are among the symptoms. You might feel tired all day long; but, thankfully, all of this is temporary and can be prevented as well. You should ensure proper hydration to prevent the severe symptoms.

Drinking adequate water is a very important part of the diet, and more so during the period of adaptation. Dehydration will worsen the symptoms. Adding a bit of salt will also help; however, you may experience some painful cramps in the legs as well. These can be a cause of real discomfort, as they occur during the day at any time and even while you are sleeping.

Drinking plenty of water will cause you to urinate often and that will cause the body to lose minerals. This is why there could be cramps in the arms. But as long as you keep drinking water with a pinch of salt, the problem will subside. You should also consider having magnesium supplements if it is too much, but they are generally not necessary.

Dehydration, mineral loss due to frequent urination, and the introduction of more dairy products in the diet may also cause constipation. Constipation is in fact most generally felt during the first stage. Constipation can be very unhealthy to the body, and consult the doctor if it does not pass soon. Assure that the body is supplied with adequate food and liquids to help regulate bowel movements.

Enhanced ketone output due to ketosis will also induce breathing by acetone. Bad breath is one of the most noticeable symptoms you're going to have to deal with so try to keep a few mints on you. Just make sure you practice good oral hygiene, so it doesn't turn into a serious problem. Some people have also noticed the heart palpitations and shakiness they experience. Diarrhea may be a part of the experience as well. It's normal to see that your sugar cravings decrease, but at the beginning of the diet, your physical performance does so.

You should consider adding additional mineral supplements to your diet to help with these symptoms. Sodium, potassium, or magnesium should be in these. Doctors or dietitians can be contacted to help you make the transition easier. They'll guide you to take the steps necessary to prevent these symptoms. Please note that all these side effects are temporary, they disappear after a while, so for a few days you just have to tolerate it. Hopefully it gets better and in reality the diet should help you become more balanced and safer.

What causes Keto flu is the metabolic change that takes place when you turn from the usual diet to the Carnivore Diet. You may experience symptoms such as nausea, cramps, night sweats, chills, dry mouth, headaches, dizziness, sleeplessness and digestive problems. Your energy level is going to be low and you may feel brain fog too.

The carnivorous diet helps trigger ketosis in your body to help you lose weight. When that happens, the body starts burning fats instead of glucose for energy. While this transformation is happening, the body will undergo three significant changes. Therefore, the fluids inside the body will be rebalanced.

The insulin level in your body reduces since the diet removes carbohydrates. Because of this insulin drop, the kidneys remove sodium in your body from water. Because of this, the first initial weight loss at the start of the diet is just water weight being lost. Then the body begins to drain its glycogen storage and after that, fats are consumed for energy gain.

Furthermore, instead of sugars the body turns to burning fats for energy. Your body is now used to burning sugars to get energy for glucose. It will start burning fats from your food as well as the accumulated fat in your body when you start the Carnivore Diet, and use this as the main source of energy. Every individual in the source of energy will respond to this switch differently.

If your body is able to handle the transition well, you will not experience symptoms of Keto flu or at least not too many; but, if this change is more difficult for your body to cope with, you will feel the pain that Keto flu can cause. If you're someone in your diet who typically eats tons of carbohydrates, your body is used to using them for energy. This is why changing the body can take longer than some others who might not be as carb reliant as you are. Indeed, cutting off carbs from your diet may even feel similar to trying to cut off caffeine or nicotine addictions.

Second, there is a biochemical reequilibrium. In this process the amount of cortisol and thyroid hormone in your body will be subject to some changes. At this stage, the thyroid hormone or T3 level in the body will diminish as it is influenced by a person's carbohydrate consumption. Such hormones will also influence body temperature changes, heart rate and the metabolism.

Dealing with the symptoms

It is important to take some steps to address certain symptoms. Such measures will either allow you to avoid any symptoms entirely, or at least reduce their effect on your body.

Hydration

The consumption of adequate water is one of the most important steps you need to take. It's also the easiest to follow to stay hydrated so don't forget this suggestion. When adopting the Carnivore Diet, ensure that you drink at least 8 glasses a day. Water is something you can take just as often as possible. As you already know, bottled juices or sodas are not allowed, so water is only your choice. Black tea and coffee are allowed but only to a point.

The diet will affect the body with a diuretic effect and this will cause a lot of loss of electrolytes. To replenish this you have to continually hydrate. Since insulin levels are also dropping during this diet, the body can excrete even more salts. The salt lost must be replenished to a safe level. Just like the cravings of sugar, you may sometimes feel like you are craving something salty. It's the way your body asks you to replenish the missing salt.

Drinking plenty of water will in many ways help you. It will help to flush out toxins from your body and will also make your skin much smoother. A high intake of sugar and carb has a negative effect on the skin, and often causes acne. Adequate Carnivore Diet hydration can help counteract on this. If you don't have the habit of drinking enough water already, set a reminder to help you get out first.

Try to drink a glass of water just about every hour. Add some electrolytes to it, if you want. Some people like to add natural flavors such as lemon, cucumber or mint leaves to make them drink more water, too. Typically such beverages are called detox water because the added ingredients contribute antioxidants to the body. Adding some flavour is an easy way to hydrate yourself.

Drink a glass of water approximately 30 minutes before each meal you enjoy. You should also make the drinking of water as easy as possible for yourself. If you're going around a lot, simply bring with you a water sipper or bottle. It must be handy to ensure you don't forget to drink water. Remember to stay away from any sweetened drinks even if it is labeled as health drinks.

If you're drinking coffee outside, choose an Americano, not a Frappuccino. Try and set a target for regular drinking water. There are a number of different ways to keep track of your water intake and keep you motivated. You can keep a diary, or simply download some software built for this very purpose.

Positivity

Positivity will play a major role while you're following the diet and overall in your life. Don't expect immediate results, and don't allow yourself to be demotivated. Within a few weeks the body becomes adapted and begins to show positive dietary effects. You should also remember that the number on the weight scale is not always the one that makes a difference. You may be burning fat but gaining muscle, so that number may not change much; however, you may try to keep track of your body measurements that are more likely to change.

The fat around your stomach regions, buttocks, etc. will decrease and thus your body size will change. Use these improvements as a reason to see more effects and be patient. When you carry on adopting the diet for long enough, you will be pleasantly surprised. Also, pictures are a great way to keep motivated and track the changes. At every stage of the diet you can compare the photos and see for yourself how your body has changed for the better.

Stress management is important to deal with stress. This can be a real impediment to physical and psychological wellbeing. Stress will even hamper your body's cycle of causing ketosis, and affect how much fat you will consume. There is a natural tendency, as stress levels increase in the body, to crave comfort foods that typically come in the form of sugar or carb-laden foods. This will encourage you to break off the diet and indulge in unhealthy food which will once again raise your weight. You've got to learn stress management to stop all of this. There are various methods, such as meditation or just some hobby, that will help you do this. Higher levels of stress make for better wellbeing.

WHY PLANTS ARE ELIMINATED ON THE CARNIVORE DIET

You may be curious about the rationale behind doing away with all plant foods from your diet. You've probably heard for years that a plant-based diet is your healthiest choice, and also the best bet for weight loss. The common assumption is that the more fruit and vegetables you consume, the better you are going to be; but were you aware of the fact that almost all of the processed food you eat is plant based? Trust us when we say this, for it's real. Do you still think all vegetable-based foods are healthy? We do not overlook the fact that for some people a plant-based diet works pretty well, but for some others it is not the case.

Each individual has a different and unique pattern of genetic makeup, immune system and microbiome. The basic biology is the same, so everyone believes that what works for one person should work for the other as well; however, the biochemical structure is completely different and not the same as the basic anatomy itself. The plant foods you eat might be a cause of your body's inflammation, digestive problems and even hormonal imbalances.

Whether you suffer from metabolic problems or leaky gut, this can also be attributed to plant-sourced so-called "organic" foods. Therefore, it is not acceptable to say generically that plant foods are good for everyone. These generalization about people who are actually negatively affected by plant compounds can be deceptive and even harmful.

There's a lot of diets out there that people randomly adopt without doing the proper research. Most of these advocate fat or carbs exclusion, and encourage you to consume as many fruits or vegetables as possible. One such form of fad diet includes a cycle of cleansing which is achieved by drinking only green smoothies. You can eat no solid foods and mix all the green ingredients into a smoothie as a replacement for your dinner. There was a case of a woman adopting the diet published in a popular medical journal in America. Due to that diet, this woman ended up having acute kidney failure.

We're not trying to prove green vegetables are hazardous to everyone. You don't even have to stop drinking green smoothies; however, the argument is that while such a diet may have benefited one person who prescribed it to that woman, it has had a very negative impact on her life. Each food can have an inverse effect on one person's body even if it has a positive effect on another.

In such cases it may be difficult to identify exactly what causes an unpleasant symptom in your body. If you're eating a variety of foods in your diet, the main aggravator is hard to identify. It could be just one particular type of vegetable that's harmful to you. A lot of people have used the carnivorous diet as a help to define those.

Tracking the attacker not only helps, but an all-meat diet has also been effective in preventing health problems. The Carnivore Diet has also helped restore hormonal balance to a more stable system. That's why we're trying to explain why all meat going is going to benefit you and why plants aren't always perfect as they are made to be.

We always have reasons among the majority of vegetarians to rationalize why they choose not to eat meat, and why others should do the same. Another such argument is that eating meat is a form of animal cruelty and this also extends to the use of all items related to animals. It is a violation of this right that all living creatures have equal right to live and we should not kill them for food.

We all say that if everyone stopped eating meat, all animals would live in peace and that would make the world a better place; but, if you use the claim of living creatures, you have to remember that all plants are living creatures as well. Why are animals more entitled to life than plants? Plants will ideally be avoided since they cannot protect themselves in any way whatsoever.

On the other side, animals have their own way of defending themselves from other predators as well as from humans. The only way plants can defend themselves is when they are being consumed. This is when their compounds are going to react with your body, causing inflammation, autoimmune disorders, pain, and some may even kill. We all know certain plant types can be poisonous if ingested.

Plants can produce a number of anti-nutrients or toxins that harm your body. Most people are totally ignorant about this negative aspect and concentrate only on how much nutrients a plant has, or what its advantages are. You'd be surprised to learn that it includes widely eaten plants such as tomatoes, onions, eggplants and even goji berries among those that cause inflammation.

Seeds are considered superfoods but they usually contain an anti-nutrient called phytic acid. The phytic acid can also be present in grains and legumes. It impacts the body's absorption of minerals such as zinc, iron, and calcium. Green leafy vegetables are also commonly promoted as superfoods in a healthy diet, but they contain oxalates which some bodies cannot process. This may be a source of oxidative stress and chronic pain if the oxalate is not digested.

Additionally, lectin in grains and legumes can be a cause for health problems. This component induces leaky intestinal conditions, autoimmune conditions and also increases inflammation. Lectin changes your body's microbiome system too.

A number of insecticides, chemicals, etc. are used to help in the process as plants are being grown. These chemicals contain salicylates which build up over time in the human body. High levels of this compound are a source of ulcers and tinnitus in the body. Usually the main plant foods in our body which increase salicylates include grapes, avocados, honey, berries, dry fruits and even spices. Do you eat a lot of crunchy vegetables like broccoli, cabbage or kale? These are a common component of diets for weight loss; however they contain goitrogens that can be very harmful to your body's thyroid hormone level.

As you can see, there are numerous harmful ingredients in different plants that can wreak havoc on your body. Many of these can cause some serious health problems and are evidently not healthy for you even if they are for someone else. Do not believe all plants are bad for everyone and should be eliminated from your diet forever; however, you must be mindful that everything has its good and bad side.

Like anything else this applies to plant foods. Do not believe eating a lot of plants in your diet would guarantee good health and longevity. For some it might be and for others it won't. All this knowledge will likely remove any reservations about following the Carnivore Diet right now. You can understand why there's so many benefits to eliminating plants from your diet and changing to a short-term all-meat diet at least. Long-term goings will depend on their impact on your body and your personal choice.

CHAPTER 7: CARNIVORE DIET FOOD CHOICES

Eating meat and sometimes other animal-sourced food is the basic guideline for a carnivorous diet. There is no other rule to this diet you need to think about. It doesn't matter what time you eat, how much you consume, what the portion size is, or even what the macronutrient amount is. Eat just when you feel hungry, and eat meat only. We will clarify any doubts about what you can eat in this section and also help you get an understanding of how you can plan your breakfast lunch or dinner according to the Carnivore Diet.

Meat

The usual source of food in this diet is meat from diverse animals. You can eat red meat such as beef, pork, wild game, lamb or even bird's meat. The diet includes all meat options, but beef is the most preferred one. You can also eat chicken or turkey white meat. It involves fish or other seafood such as new oysters, lobster, crab, shrimp, and squid. Organ meat is also allowed so you may consume the liver, bone marrow, heart, brain or kidney of any animal.

Also eggs are a good source of protein in this diet and can come from chickens, geese or ducks. Don't just try to eat only lean meat, even include the fatty cuts in your diet. The meat fat provides your daily nutritional needs. This will also provide the protein, minerals, and other nutrients you need. The fatty meat cuts will help make your diet more palatable.

We'll give you the best cuts and types to choose from amongst the meat options you have. You can eat lamb chops, ribs or shanks, if you like beef. Wings, thighs and drumsticks are all good for poultry. Select meat from the neck, ribs, butt roast or pork belly, in the case of pork. Fish gives you lots of options including salmon, shrimp, trout, scallops, sardines, mackerel and crab. Of any of the species you can also have bone broth.

You may wonder if consuming grass-fed meat is just as important. While this would be your healthiest option, it's understandable that it's more costly, too. Don't let this bother you too much, and choose meats within your budget. The high grass-fed meat costs shouldn't deter you from beginning a Carnivore Diet. When it comes to processed meat, avoid these at least during the first 30 days of trying the Carnivore Diet. That will make the diet more effective and safer for you. You should eat sausages, but avoid bacon.

Animal meat is recommended in the carnivorous diet because it contains DHA, and this will help improve brain function. Including or removing offal from your diet is a personal choice.

Dairy

Some foods are listed in the "maybe" category. They may be available in minimum quantities on occasion but not regularly or in large quantities. These are technically sourced from animals, so they don't defy the guidelines completely, but they're still not meat. These include dairy products such as heavy cream, butter, ghee, milk, yogurt, and cheese; however, most people prefer not to eat dairy particularly if they want to lose weight more quickly. This is largely due to the fact that dairy contains lactose, and should be limited even if eaten.

Coffee, tea and coffee

Water is your natural drink and should be preferred to stay hydrated over anything else, no matter what diet you adopt. Coffee and tea, while plant-sourced, are exceptions to the limitations on a diet. The only rule is to get them plain, with no sugar or additives. Such two ingredients do have many advantages on their own and even act as a natural insecticide. It can be difficult for people to adapt to the Carnivore Diet if they also have to adapt to the withdrawal of caffeine at the same time; however, once you're adjusted to the diet, try cutting your caffeine habit too.

The only taste enhancers permitted are salt and pepper and these should also be used within a cap. Spices are, in truth, another exception to the law, not stressed as much. It's also advised to remove these from the diet, but you can choose to use some in your food for added flavour. Try not to overdo it. Turmeric is one of the beneficial spices that should be considered because it helps in immunity and also improves the health of the cognitive and brain. Cayenne pepper has particular advantages in the weight loss process.

Herbs are not only flavourful but have many health benefits as well. Including some of these to your meat-based meals will help improve your health as well as add a variety of tastes to this restrictive diet. Cinnamon is one of those helpful herbs that adds spice and controls blood sugar levels as well. Actually it acts as a kind of natural insulin. Oregano is another herb that gets infused with flavour. This contains lots of antioxidants and combines well with various flavours. Rosemary should also be considered as it helps to reduce inflammation in your body. Inflammation is one of the major causes of arthritis, and the associated risk may be reduced by rosemary. Thyme is high in antioxidants and is important for safe breathing.

Supplements

Usually, you wouldn't need any additional supplements; however, some people do need them, and during the adaptation period they may need them. Allowed supplements include Himalayan salt, electrolytes, and lipase or Ox bile for GI support; however, these are cut off after the period of adaptation has passed.

Let's see what a day looks like in terms of your meals on the Carnivore Diet.

Breakfast

You can eat a few eggs in the morning which can be cooked or boiled in butter. This meal can also be served with cheese and ham. If you want a coffee or tea, make it black.

Lunch

In the afternoon, go ahead and have a steak with a rib eye. You can also have other cuts of beef, such as sirloin, strip or chuck eye. Go for a roast if you don't want a steak. It will seem like a dream come true for those who had to stop that on a different diet before.

Dinner

Your dinner may be a hamburger patty with some cooked bacon. If the lack of buns makes you feel dissatisfied, you can even have an extra patty. Instead of the patties you can also opt for a T-bone steak.

We recommend abstaining from snacks because meat is very filling and this is easy. This leaves you much more comfortable and you'll rarely feel hungry until your next meal is ready. If you're still hungry all the time, consider increasing the fatty cuts in your meals, because they're more filling. Consider some pork rinds when you desperately need a snack.

Foods to avoid while on the Carnivore Diet

On the Carnivore Diet you almost have to stop eating anything that doesn't fall into the meat category. This includes:

- Vegetables

- Fruit

- Nuts

- Legumes

- Grains

- Pasta

- Rice

- Seasonings or sauces

- Processed meat

- No vegetable oils

Avoid any processed meats such as bacon, salami, pepperoni or chorizo. These are the carbohydrate fillers, which should be avoided particularly on this diet; but, if you can stick to the best possible diet in the first month, you can sometimes enjoy these processed meats as snacks later. If you are traveling these may be your best option to stick to the diet; however, try to avoid as much as possible anything that's processed.

Stop buying sausages prepared beforehand. These typically contain wheat which is added to fill out the sausage. At home, you can try and make your own healthy ones. Don't buy in-market sausages or hotdogs off the stand. These will affect the diet, and can also lead to weight gain.

CARNIVORE DIET BREAKFAST RECIPES

1. Simple Boiled Eggs

Serves: 2

Ingredients:

- 4 eggs

- Water, as required

- Salt to taste (optional)

- Pepper to taste (optional)

Method:

Half fill a pan with water and place over high heat. When water begins to boil, lower the heat to low heat. Carefully lower the eggs into the pan. Cook until the desired temperature depending on the size of the eggs.

For soft-boiled eggs: Let the eggs cook for 4-5 minutes.

For medium boiled eggs: Let the eggs cook for 7-8 minutes.

For hard- boiled eggs: Cook for 8-10 minutes.

Drain and place in a bowl of chilled water.

Peel after 4-5 minutes.

Season with salt and pepper if desired and serve.

2. Fried Eggs

Serves: 2

Ingredients:

- 4 eggs

- Salt to taste

- Pepper to taste

- 4 teaspoons butter

Method:

Place a nonstick pan over medium heat. Add 1-teaspoon butter and melt. Crack an egg into the pan.

Cook until the whites are set and the yolk is runny. Remove with a spatula on to a plate.

For over-easy: When the whites are set, flip side once. Cook for about 30 seconds and remove on to a plate.

For over- medium: When the whites are set, flip side once. Cook for about 1 – 1-½ minutes.

For over-hard: When the whites are set, flip side once. Cook for 2-3 minutes or until the yolk is cooked well, as in a hard- boiled egg.

For steam-fried eggs: Cook the eggs, sunny side up (step 2) but cover the pan with a lid when the whites are lightly set.

Cook the remaining eggs following step 1 and 2 /3/4/5/6

Season with salt and pepper and serve.

3. Soft and Creamy Scrambled Eggs

Serves: 1

Ingredients:

- 2 large free-range eggs

- 1 teaspoon butter

- Salt to taste

- Freshly cracked pepper to taste (optional)

Method:

Crack eggs into a bowl. Add and salt and whisk lightly until well combined.

Place a nonstick pan over medium heat. Add butter and let it melt. Add the egg mixture. Do not stir for 20 seconds.

Using a silicone spatula, stir lightly in small circles for the initial 30 seconds, until slightly curdled.

Stir in bigger circles for the next 15 to 20 seconds the egg is curdy in texture. The eggs should be soft and yet set and runny in a few places.

Turn off the heat. Let it cook in the heat for 8-10 seconds.

Stir lightly. Season with pepper and more salt if desired and serve immediately.

4. Perfect Scrambled Eggs

Serves: 2

Ingredients:

- 4 large free-range eggs

- 4 tablespoons butter

- ¾ cup single cream or full cream milk

- Salt to taste

- Pepper to taste (optional)

Method:

Whisk together eggs in a bowl. Add cream or milk, pepper and salt and whisk until well combined.

Place a nonstick pan over medium heat. Add butter. When butter melts, add the egg mixture. Do not stir for 20 seconds.

Stir lightly using a wooden spoon. Lift and fold the egg over from the bottom of the pan.

Do not stir for another 10 seconds. Lift and fold the egg over from the bottom of the pan.

Repeat the previous step until the eggs are cooked soft, but also runny at different spots. Turn off the heat.

Stir lightly one last time and serve immediately.

5. Individual Baked Eggs

Serves: 2

Ingredients:

- 2 slices bacon

- 2 eggs

- ½ slice cheddar cheese, cut into 2 halves (in other words two pieces of ¼ slice cheese)

- 2 teaspoons melted butter

Method:

Place a deep skillet over medium-high heat. Add cook until brown, yet soft and workable.

Remove bacon and put on a plate lined with paper towels.

Take 2 muffin cups. Line the inside of each muffin cup with a slice of bacon.

Put a teaspoon of butter in each cup.

Crack an egg into each cup.

Bake in a preheated oven at 350° about F for 10-15 minutes depending on how you like it cooked.

Place a piece of cheese on top. Bake for some more time until cheese melts.

Serve hot.

6. Scotch Eggs

Serves: 3

Ingredients:

● 3 medium eggs

● ¼ teaspoon salt or to taste

● ½ pound ground or minced pork or beef or lamb or chicken, preferably lean meat

● Pepper to taste (optional)

Method:

Half fill a pan with some water and place over high heat. When water begins to boil, lower the heat to low heat. Carefully lower the eggs into the pan.

Let the eggs cook for 4 minutes.

Drain and place in a bowl of chilled water.

Peel after 4-5 minutes. Dry the eggs by patting with kitchen towels.

Add meat (it is better to use lean meat, as the meat may fall apart while baking), salt and pepper into a bowl and mix well. Divide the mixture into 3 equal portions.

Take one portion of meat, place on your palm and flatten it. Place one egg in the center and bring the edges together to enclose the egg. Place on a baking sheet, greased with butter.

Repeat with the remaining meat and eggs.

Bake in a preheated oven at about 350° F for 30 minutes depending on how you like it cooked.

7. Eggs Lorraine

Serves: 1

Ingredients:

- 2 slices Canadian bacon

- 2 eggs

- Salt to taste

- 1 slice Swiss cheese

- 1 tablespoon sour cream

- Pepper to taste

Method:

Take a shallow, oval shaped baking dish (of about 1 ½ cups capacity) cups. Line the inside dish with a bacon. Place a cheese slice in the dish.

Crack the eggs into the dish.

Add sour cream, salt and pepper into a bowl and mix well. Pour into the baking dish.

Bake in a preheated oven at about 350° F for 10-15 minutes, until the eggs are cooked.

Serve hot.

8. Chicken and Bacon Sausage

Serves: 24

Ingredients:

- 4 large chicken breasts or 2 pounds ground chicken

- 2 eggs, beaten

- 4 slices bacon, cooked, crumbled

- Salt to taste

- Pepper to taste

Method:

Add all the ingredients in the food processor bowl. Process until well combined.

Divide the mixture into 24 equal portions and shape into patties of about ½ inch thickness.

Place the patties on a baking tray lined with foil.

Bake in a preheated oven at 425° F for 20-25 minutes depending on how you like it cooked.

Remove from the oven and cool completely. It can be frozen or refrigerated until use.

CARNIVORE DIET SNACK RECIPES

1. Devilled Eggs

Serves: 2

Ingredients:

- 4 eggs

- Water, as required

- Salt or Himalayan pink salt to taste

- Pepper to taste (optional)

- 2 tablespoons crumbled cheese

Method:

Half fill a saucepan with water and place over high heat. When water begins to boil, lower the heat to low heat. Carefully lower the eggs into the pan. Cook for 8-10 minutes.

Drain and place in a bowl of chilled water.

Peel after 4-5 minutes.

Halve the eggs lengthwise. Carefully scoop the yolks from the eggs and place in a bowl.

Add salt, pepper and cheese and mash well. Fill the mixture into the cavity of the yolks with a spoon or transfer the mixture into a piping bag and pipe it into the cavities.

Serve as it is or chill and serve later.

2. Meatballs

Serves: 4-5

Ingredients:

- 2 1/4 pounds ground beef

- 1 teaspoon salt

- 6 tablespoons, grated parmesan cheese

- 1 teaspoon pepper

Method:

Add all the ingredients inside a bowl and mix until well combined.

Make small balls of the mixture and place on a lined baking sheet.

Bake in a preheated oven at about 350 ° F for about 20-30 minutes depending on the size of the meatballs. Turn the balls around a couple of times while baking.

Alternately, place the meatballs in a skillet and cover with a lid. Cook until done. Turn the balls around a couple of times.

3. Cheese and Meat Roll Ups

Serves: 4

Ingredients:

- 4 slices cooked turkey

- 4 slices cheese

Method:

Place turkey slices on a serving platter. Place a slice of cheese on each. Roll and place with the seam sides facing down. Fasten with toothpick if desired and serve.

4. Pepperoni Meatballs

Serves: 8

Ingredients:

- 2 pounds ground beef or chicken

- 1 teaspoon salt or to taste

- 1 teaspoon pepper or to taste

- 2 eggs, whisked

- ½ pound pepperoni slices, ground or minced

Method:

Add all the ingredients inside a mixing bowl and mix until well combined.

Make small balls of the mixture and place on a lined baking sheet.

Bake in a preheated oven at about 350 ° F for about 20-30 minutes depending on the size of the meatballs. Turn the balls around a couple of times while baking.

Alternately, place the meatballs in a skillet and cover with a lid. Cook until done. Turn the balls around a couple of times.

5. Liver Burgers

Serves: 7-8

Ingredients:

- 1 pound grass fed beef

- ½ teaspoon pepper

- ½ pound ground liver, drain excess mixing blood

Method:

Add all the ingredients into a bowl and mix using your hands.

Make 7-8 equal portions of the mixture and shape into patties.

Grill on a preheated gill on both the sides until the desired doneness is achieved and serve.

CARNIVORE DIET SOUP AND BROTH RECIPES

1. Japanese Tonkotsu Ramen Broth

Serves: 8

Ingredients:

- 1 ¼ pounds pork bones, without any meat

- 1 ¼ pounds pig trotters, only leg portion

- Bones of 1 whole chicken

- 5 1/3 ounces pork skin (optional)

- 8 quarts water + extra to blanch

Method:

Chop the larger bones into smaller pieces.

To blanch the bones: Take a large pot. Place trotters and all the bones in it. Pour enough water to cover the bones.

Place the pot over medium heat. Bring to a boil. Boil for 10 minutes. Remove from heat. Pour out the water and then rinse the pot well. Remove the bones and keep it aside.

Clean the bones of any blood clots with a sharp knife.

Add the bones back to the pot with the pork skin. Add 8 quarts of water to it. Bring to a boil.

Lower heat and let it simmer.

Initially scum will start floating. Remove the scum with a large spoon and discard. Trim the excess fat too.

Cover and simmer for about 12- 15 hours. The stock would have reduced in quantity and will be thicker.

Remove from heat. When it cools down, strain into a large jar with a wire mesh strainer.

Refrigerate for 5-6 days. Unused broth can be frozen.

Heat thoroughly, then serve.

2. Iced Bone Broth

Serves:

Ingredients:

- 2 pounds bones, preferably with a little meat on them

- Water, as required

- Himalayan pink salt to taste

Method:

Place bones in a pot. Fill the pot with water (at least 5 quarts). Add 1-teaspoon salt.

Place the pot over medium heat. Bring to a boil. Boil for 5 minutes. Cover with a lid. Lower the heat and simmer for 4-5 hours.

When the broth is ready, remove the meat if any and use.

Strain the broth and cool completely. Use as required.

For iced broth: Fill glasses with crushed ice. Pour broth into the glasses and serve.

Pour leftovers in a jar and refrigerate until use.

3. Bacon Cheeseburger Soup

Serves: 2

Ingredients:

- ½ pound ground beef

- 2 cups bone broth

- Salt to taste

- Pepper to taste (optional)

- ¼ cup heavy cream

- ¼ cup bacon bits

- ½ cup milk

- 1 cup cheddar cheese, shredded

Method:

Place a soup pot over medium heat. Add the bacon then cook it until brown and crisp.

Add beef and cook until brown. Break it simultaneously as it cooks.

Stir in the broth, milk, salt and pepper.

When it starts to boil, reduce the heat and simmer for 8-10 minutes.

Turn off the heat. Add cheese and cream and stir until cheese melts completely.

Ladle into soup bowls and serve.

4. Creamy Chicken Soup

Serves: 8

Ingredients:

- 4 tablespoons butter

- 8 ounces cream cheese, cubed

- 4 cup chicken bone broth

- Salt to taste

- Pepper to taste

- 4 cups cooked, shredded chicken breast

- ½ cup heavy cream

Method:

Place a saucepan over medium heat. Add butter and butter melt. Add chicken and sauté for a couple of minutes until the chicken is well coated with the butter.

Add cream cheese and mix well.

When cream cheese melts, add broth and cream and stir.

Add salt and pepper and stir.

Ladle into soup bowls and serve.

5. Cheddar Chicken Soup

Serves: 8

Ingredients:

- 1 pound chicken breasts, skinless, boneless, chopped into bite size chunks

- 4 cups milk

- 2 cups shredded cheddar cheese

- 6 cups chicken broth

- Salt to taste

- 1 tablespoon butter

Method:

Place a saucepan over medium heat. Add butter and butter melt. Add chicken and sauté for a couple of minutes until the chicken is well coated with the butter.

Stir in the broth and milk. Cook until chicken is tender.

Turn off the heat.

Add cheese and salt and stir it until cheese melts.

Ladle into soup bowls and serve.

CARNIVORE DIET POULTRY RECIPES

1. Salt and Pepper Turkey

Serves: 5-8

Ingredients:

- 1 whole turkey of about 9-10 pounds, discard giblets

- 3-5 tablespoons butter

- Coarse salt to taste

- Freshly ground pepper to taste

Method:

Pour 2 cups water in a large roasting pan. Place a rack in the pan.

Start at the neck and loosen the skin on the breast area. Take some of the butter and rub it beneath the skin.

Sprinkle salt and pepper, generously all over the turkey and the cavity. Using a thick kitchen string, tie up the legs together. Place turkey on the rack and tuck the wings below.

Bake in a preheated oven at 350 ° F for 2-3 hours or until the internal temperature when checked with an instant reading thermometer in the thickest part of the meat shows 165 ° F.

Baste the turkey with remaining butter after every 25 to 30 minutes. Slightly shake the turkey so that the cooked juice falls into the pan.

Remove turkey from the oven and place on your cutting board. Cover with foil and then let it sit for 30 minutes.

When cool enough to handle, cut into slices. Drizzle some of the cooked liquid from the pan over the turkey and serve.

2. Turkey in Cream Sauce

Serves: 4

Ingredients:

- 3 tablespoons butter

- ¾ cup heavy cream

- Salt to taste

- Pepper to taste

- ¾ cup chicken stock

- 2 cups cooked, chopped turkey

Method:

Place a large pan over medium heat. Add butter and cook until it turns brown or golden in color.

Add stock and simmer for 5-6 minutes.

Add cream, turkey, salt and pepper. Simmer for a few minutes.

Serve hot.

3. Duck Leg Confit

Serves: 2

Ingredients:

- 2 duck legs with thigh, trimmed of excess fat and retain it

- 3-5 tablespoons butter

- Table salt to taste

- ½ tablespoon kosher salt

- Freshly ground pepper to taste

- 2 cups duck fat (that was retained)

- ¾ teaspoon whole peppercorns

Method:

Place the duck legs on a large plate, with the skin side facing down. Season with kosher salt and pepper.

Pour the duck fat in a baking dish.

Stack the duck legs in the baking dish and place in the refrigerator for 10 to 12 hours.

Remove the duck and rinse in cold water. Lightly wipe off the salt and pepper.

Dry with paper towels.

Remove the duck fat and place in an enameled cast iron pot.

Scatter peppercorns on the fat. Sprinkle salt over it.

Place the duck, with the skin side facing down in the pot. Place some duck fat on top of the duck. Cover and place in a preheated oven.

Bake at 350 ° F for about 2-3 hours or until the meat falls away from the bone.

Strain the fat from the dish into a bowl. Retain the fat to store meat or use in some other recipe.

If you want serve right away, transfer the duck legs into a pan, with the skin side facing down. Place the pan over medium high heat and sear until the skin is crisp and brown.

If you want to eat after a few days, remove the meat from the bones and keep it in a stoneware container. Pour some of the retained fat over the meat. (Fat should cover by at least ¼ inch over the meat). Place the container in the refrigerator until use. It can last for a month.

4. BBQ Chicken Livers and Hearts

Serves: 4-6

Ingredients:

- 2 pounds chicken livers, thawed to room temperature

- 2 pounds chicken hearts, thawed to room temperature

- Pepper to taste

- Salt to taste

- A few bamboo skewers, soaked in water for an hour

Method:

Clear the excess fat from the hearts and livers and clean them too.

Place them flat, in a flexible grilling basket.

Sprinkle salt and pepper over the meat.

Grill on a charcoal grill until the way you like it cooked.

5. Chicken with Cheesy Sauce

Serves: 3

Ingredients:

- 6 chicken thighs

- ½ teaspoon pepper

- ½ teaspoon salt

- 1 cup chicken bone broth

- 4 ounces cream cheese

- ½ cup heavy cream

- 10 tablespoons butter, divided

- 1 cup mozzarella cheese, shredded

Method:

Place a large skillet over medium heat. Add two teaspoons of butter and allow it to heat.

Sprinkle salt and pepper over the chicken. Sprinkle beneath the skin also.

Place chicken in the skillet with the skin side facing down.

Cover and cook for 6 minutes or until the skin side is brown. Remove the chicken with slotted spoon and set aside on another plate.

Pour broth into the skillet. Scrape the base of the pan to get rid of any browned bits that may be stuck.

Add chicken back into the pan. Cover and cook until the chicken is cooked through.

Meanwhile, make the sauce as follows: Add cream cheese, cream and remaining butter into a saucepan. Place saucepan over low heat.

Stir constantly until the mixture is well incorporated. Turn off the heat.

Whisk in the mozzarella cheese. Stir constantly until cheese melts.

Place chicken in bowls. Pour cheesy sauce over it and serve.

6. Simple, Pan-fried Chicken Breasts

Serves: 4-

Ingredients:

- 8 chicken breast halves

- 2 tablespoons butter or lard

- Freshly ground pepper to taste

- Kosher salt to taste

- ¼ cup grated parmesan cheese (optional)

Method:

Place a stainless steel or cast – iron skillet over medium heat. Add butter or lard and let the pan heat.

Using a meat mallet, grind the chicken breast until the chicken is uniformly thick.

Season with salt and pepper if using. Let it rest for 15-20 minutes.

Place an ovenproof skillet over high heat. Place chicken in the skillet.

Cook for 2-3 minutes without stirring or covering. Cook until golden brown and the fat is released. Flip sides cook for 2-3 minutes.

Remove from the heat and garnish with desired sides, best with Parmesan cheese.

Broil for 2-3 minutes and serve.

7. Chicken with Creamy Bacon Sauce

Serves: 10

Ingredients:

- 10 chicken thighs

- ½ teaspoon pepper

- ½ teaspoon salt

- 1 cup chicken bone broth

- 1 cup double heavy cream

- 4 tablespoons butter, softened

- 16 slices bacon

Method:

Place a pan over medium heat. Add bacon and cook until brown. Drain the fat remaining in the pan. When cool enough to carry, chop into small pieces. Set aside.

Place a large skillet over medium heat. Add butter and melt.

Sprinkle salt and pepper over the chicken. Sprinkle beneath the skin as well.

Place chicken in the skillet with the skin side facing down.

Cover and cook for 6 minutes or until the skin side is brown. Remove chicken with a slotted spoon and set aside on a plate.

Pour broth into the skillet. Scrape the base of the pot to remove any browned bits that may be stuck.

Add chicken back into the pan. Add half the bacon. Cover and cook until chicken is well cooked and edible. Remove chicken with a slotted spoon and set aside.

Add cream and remaining butter into the same skillet.

Stir constantly until the mixture is well incorporated.

Add chicken back into the skillet and mix well. Simmer for a couple of minutes. Turn off the heat.

Place chicken in bowls. Sprinkle remaining bacon on top and serve.

8. Easy Chicken Salad

Serves: 4-5

Ingredients:

- 1 cup sour cream

- 4-5 chicken breast halves

- Salt to taste

- Pepper to taste

- 1 cup feta cheese, crumbled

- 4 slices bacon

- 4 hard-boiled eggs, peeled, quartered

Method:

Place the chicken in a stockpot. Cover with cold water. Sprinkle salt.

Place the stockpot over medium heat. Cook until chicken is tender. Remove the chicken with a pair of tongs and place on your cutting board. Shred or chop into pieces.

Place a pan over medium heat. Add bacon and cook until brown.

Remove with a slotted spoon and place on a plate lined with paper towels. When cool enough to handle, chop into pieces.

Add chicken, bacon, and rest of the ingredients into a bowl and fold gently.

Chill and serve.

CARNIVORE DIET MEAT (BEEF, LAMB, PORK, ETC.) RECIPES

1. Baked / Broiled Steak

Serves: 1

Ingredients:

- 1 strip loin steaks (10-12 ounces), 1½ inches thick, at room temperature

- ¼ teaspoon kosher salt

- 1 tablespoon butter or lard, melted

- Freshly ground pepper to taste (optional)

Method:

Dry the steak by patting with paper towels.

For roasting in an oven: Brush ½ tablespoon butter over the steak and rub it well into it. Sprinkle salt and pepper if using.

Place a skillet over medium heat. When the pan heats, place steak in the skillet and cook for a minute. Flip sides and cook for a minute.

Place a rack on a rimmed baking sheet.

Place steak on the rack. Place baking sheet in the oven.

Roast in a preheated oven at 375°F:

For rare: Roast for 10 minutes and internal temperature should be 120°F.

For medium: Roast for 14 minutes and internal temperature should be 145°F.

For well cooked: Roast for 18 minutes and internal temperature should be 155°F.

For broiling in an oven: After step 2, place steak in a broiling pan. You can also keep on a rack.

Place the broiling pan 6 inches away from the heating element.

For rare: Broil for 2 minutes. Flip once and broil for 2 minutes.

For medium: Broil for 4 minutes. Flip once and broil for minutes.

For well cooked: Broil for 6 minutes. Flip once and broil for 6 minutes.

Serve hot.

2. Liver Bacon Meatballs

Serves: 6

Ingredients:

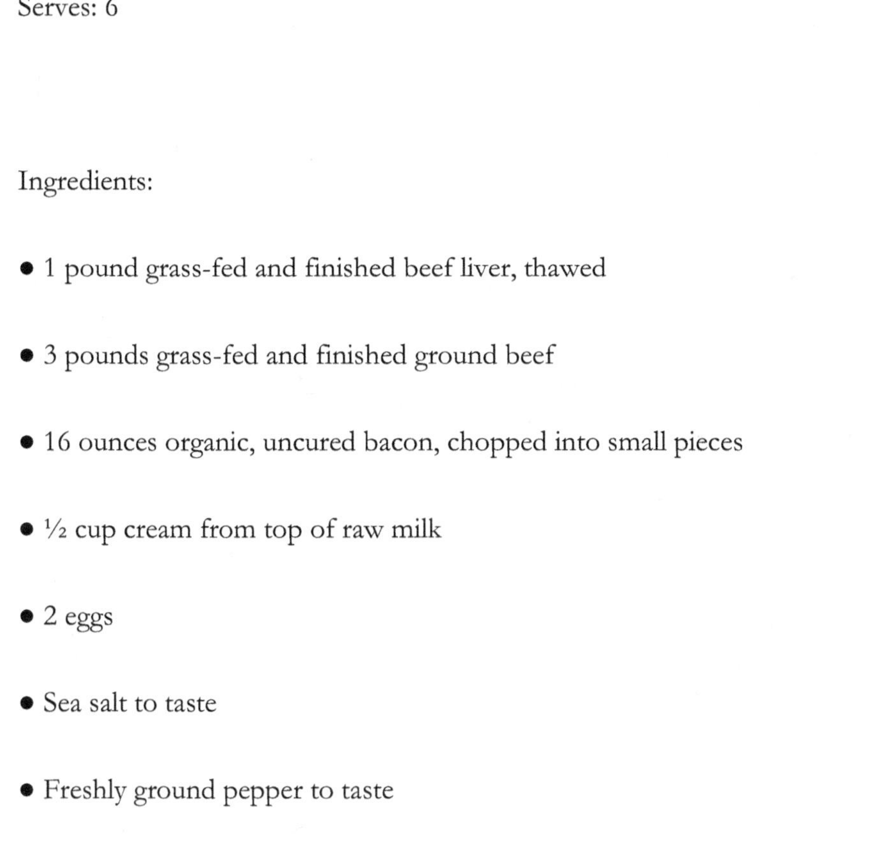

- 1 pound grass-fed and finished beef liver, thawed

- 3 pounds grass-fed and finished ground beef

- 16 ounces organic, uncured bacon, chopped into small pieces

- ½ cup cream from top of raw milk

- 2 eggs

- Sea salt to taste

- Freshly ground pepper to taste

Method:

Place a large pan over medium heat. Add bacon and cook until brown but not too crisp.

Remove bacon with a slotted spoon and place on a plate lined with layers of paper towels.

When bacon cools, transfer into the food processor bowl and process until crumbly. Add liver into the food processor bowl. Continue processing until it is liquid in texture.

Add eggs, salt, pepper and cream into a bowl and whisk well. Pour into the food processor bowl. Also add beef and pulse until well combined.

Make small balls of the mixture.

Heat the same pan in which bacon was cooked. Add meatballs and cook until brown all over (2-3 minutes on each side). Cover and cook until the meat inside is well cooked. Add more butter or lard if required will frying.

Serve hot.

3. Carnivore Burger

Serves: 8

Ingredients:

- 2 pounds ground beef

- 2 pounds ground bison

- 2 pounds ground lamb

- 2 pounds ground pork

- 8 large eggs

- Salt to taste (optional)

- Pepper to taste (optional)

Method:

Preheat grill to high heat.

Add all the meat and eggs into a large bowl and mix well using your hands.

Divide the mixture into 8 equal portions. Shape into patties of about 1 inch thickness. Season with salt and pepper if desired.

Place 2-3 burgers on the preheated grill. Grill for 5-7 minutes. Flip sides and cook for 5-7 minutes. The internal temperature of the burger should be around 135°F when checked with a meat thermometer. Grill in batches.

Remove the burgers from the grill and place on a plate. Tent with foil for 5 minutes.

Serve.

4. Carnivore Meatloaf

Serves: 2-4

Ingredients:

- 2 pounds ground pork (80/20)

- 4 pounds ground beef (80/20)

- Salt to taste

Method:

Add beef into a mixing bowl. Add salt and mix with your hands until well combined.

Add pork and knead until well combined.

Transfer into a rectangular baking dish. Press it well onto the bottom of the dish.

Bake in a preheated oven at 350°F for about 30-40 minutes or until the cooked juices are released in the center and it looks cooked at the edges. The edges will begin to leave the dish.

Remove from the oven.

Cool for a while. Cut into slices and serve.

5. Perfect Skillet Steak

Serves: 1-2

Ingredients:

- Steak of 7/8 thickness

- Butter or lard, melted, to brush

- Salt to taste

- Pepper to taste

Method:

Place a skillet over medium high heat and allow it to heat.

Brush steak with butter and place on the skillet.

For rare: Cook for 2-3 minutes. Flip sides once and cook side for 2-3 minutes. Using a pair of tongs (back part), press the steak in the center. If it is soft, turn off the heat.

For medium: Cook for 4 minutes. Flip side once and cook the other side for 4 minutes. Using a pair of tongs (back part), press the steak in the center. If it is slightly firmer, turn off the heat.

For well cooked: Cook for 5-6 minutes. Flip side once and cook the other side for 5-6 minutes. Using a pair of tongs (back part), press the steak in the center. If it is very firm, turn off the heat.

When the steak is cooked as per your liking, remove steak from the pan and place on a plate. Tent with foil and let it rest for 5 minutes.

Slice and serve. Season with salt and pepper if desired.

6. CHEESY MEATLOAF

This recipe is fun because when you cut into the meatloaf, melted cheese oozes out. It's the simple things, right?

2 pounds ground beef

¾ to 1 teaspoon sea salt, more to taste

2 eggs

5 to 7 ounces cheese, in slices, chunks, or grated

Preheat the oven to 350 degrees F.

Whisk the salt and eggs in a large bowl.

Add the beef.

Briefly mix it all together so the egg and salt is dispersed throughout the meat.

Press half of the mixture into a meatloaf baking dish.

Place the cheese as a middle layer.

Press the remaining half of beef on top of the cheese, as the top layer of the meatloaf.

Bake for about 50 minutes, depending on the internal temperature you prefer.

7. SPATCHCOCK-ROASTED CHICKEN

1 (3 to 5 pounds) whole chicken

Sea salt

Melted ghee, butter, or lard

Preheat the oven to 375 degrees F.

Spatchcock the bird: With a sharp knife, kitchen shears, or even garden shears (my preference), remove the backbone by cutting up along each side of the backbone and removing it. Save the backbone for making chicken broth.

Flip the chicken over, and split it. Spread it open and firmly press down on the chicken with both hands to flatten it. (There are many videos on YouTube.)

Generously season both sides and wings of the bird with sea salt.

Lay the bird on a baking tray, skin side up. Drizzle some animal fat on top.

Roast the bird for 45 to 60 minutes or until deepest part of the thigh reads 165 degrees F on a meat thermometer.

Transfer to a slicing let it rest for 10 to 15 minutes.

Carve and enjoy.

CHAPTER 8: FINAL NOTES

FREQUENT QUESTIONS ABOUT CARNIVORE DIET What about vitamin C, magnesium and antioxidants? Can you get these in a Carnivore Diet, and do you need them?

The idea in the carnivore community is usually that if a healthy person eats enough calories and gets all of them from beef, they should be able to get all they need from a Carnivore Diet. Some people recommend a small serve of offal, especially liver, to get a vitamin boost. Many people like Dr. Shawn Baker, though, do not take any vitamins, nor consume offal. They do not have scurvy or magnesium shortages, either.

Animal products actually absorb the vitamins and minerals faster than plant ones. That's because the fiber and the anti-nutrients (phytates) make them less bioavailable in plants.

I encountered this sad fact firsthand when I ate a vegan diet. Dr. Shawn Baker says plant-based diets push the nutrient requirements of people and make it more difficult to assimilate nutrients, because they require more transformations and more effort. Many people don't even have the organs needed to absorb many nutrients, to make matters worse. For example, consider the large portion of the population which cannot assimilate beta-carotene Vitamin A in plants. Instead, they need it in the preformed form of retinol from animal produce. That was my family and I of course.

Conversely, eating a meat-based diet decreases the nutrient requirements thus making them more bioavailable.

How much do I need to eat?

Okay, how is it that you feel hungry? A great rule of thumb for a Carnivore Diet-because eating too much is very difficult-is just letting your appetite guide you. The ease of making food choices on a Carnivore Diet can help control one's hunger and appetite. Gaining so much variety occasionally causes overeating.

That said, in the beginning, a common mistake among carnivorous newbies is simply not eating enough. They're not used to eating so much meat and therefore they don't eat enough. Energy levels are marginally increasing. As Dr. Shawn Baker is known to say, "Eat meat like it's your work." A shift tip: if you're not yet ready for a full carnivorous diet, you may first eat meat at a meal, then try to eat enough to be satisfied. Afterwards, should I drink coffee or tea on a Carnivore Diet, will you eat a few plants to top off?

Coffee is a non-carb, zero calorie plant extract. It should be looked upon as a drink, not a meal. Many carnivorous dietitians also drink coffee. I drink some coffee, but preferably only the days I'm writing or driving. I want more in cold months, too, so for me, it's a little seasonal coffee intake.

One great help in reducing coffee consumption is drinking bone broth, especially under cold weather. Broth doesn't have caffeine but it's tasty, nutritious and relaxing.

What should I eat at the Restaurants?

When I learn that I'm going to a restaurant I'm trying to find the menu online beforehand. Maybe I could also call and ask questions, as mentioned below, to arrange things before I come in.

I choose the meat dishes I'd like to see on the menu. Instead, I ask the server what they would charge for a meat-only dish.

For example, if a restaurant has a burger, then I will ask for a patty price only. If they come back with a lower price than I would pay for the whole kit (bun, condiments, sides) then yay! I shall order two or three of those patties.

But if they don't offer a cheaper price just for the patty versus getting the sandwich, and so on, I'll wonder if they can make a deal for me to get three patties alone. When I increase the number of patties and say I don't want any bun or sides, they are more prepared to come down on the price per patty.

Sometimes in a restaurant there's a big steak so I'll just order it and forget about the sides that come with the steak or tell them to leave the sides off.

Will kids eat a Carnivore Diet?

As normal, just check with your doctor. The saying is true to you, and more so to your family. As one thing their bodies continue to evolve and their needs vary from those of adults. Yet kids may also not be as attuned to what they "see" as right or wrong. You have had many years of experience and you are still not rising up. You might not know whether something is shifting to alert you, either.

Children on medical ketogenic diets have a greater chance of getting kidney stones, it has been stated. The Carnivore Diet isn't the same as the keto diet, so it's unclear if it's valid. Speak to your kid's doctor about this. And if a doctor prescribes a safe keto diet for your child, you may wonder whether, or should be, the ketogenic diet is meat-based or plant-free.

Some "experts" on carnivorous diets (including doctors) say yes, carnivorous diets for children are safe and healthy. It might be unrealistic to expect kids to always stick to it though. The children also eat carnivores inside the house in some carnivore households, and when they eat plants outside the house for warmth and social norms (i.e. parties, etc.).

One cautionary note: Many non-normal diets (and lifestyles) have a long history of spooking officials, which are understandably cautious in dealing with unknowns and child welfare. It's their job and I don't hold it against them because there are some dangerous people out there. But this means the authorities seem to be suspicious of anything that is not officially supported by the usual Three Letter Acronym authorities or the relevant government departments. When authorities obtain a carnivorous diet report or complaint about an infant, they may need to investigate legally and may feel compelled to intervene. Skip, at your own risk posting on social media that is at very high risk.

One thing I'm going to say is to let your kids eat the meat. And, probably more. And less food-dependent carbohydrate, if they are already eating a lot. Those proposals aren't controversial enough to cause concern for anyone.

Meat also gets heavily discounted just before big holidays, so it's a perfect time to stock up. Another option is to work with a local rancher, or contract a half or quarter cow directly with a local processor.

Different cuttings of meat lend themselves to different cooking techniques.

The various slow-cooking and low-temperature methods will make some of the leaner cuts very tender. Ground beef is often cheap and a delectable option. Animal meat appears to be very cost-friendly, and is likely to provide more protein per dollar than any food.

Get to know the local butcher and you can possibly get some great deals. Some butchers throw away things— like trimmed fats, organs, and bones that you can use to make broth or cook with — free.

The inclusion of eggs in your meals is another cost-effective way to supplement your diet. Eggs are often affordably priced.

Cooking methods

This book's scope does not allow for a cooking course but I have some general comments. Cooking is an essential skill, and learning how to cook a decent steak properly is especially crucial. There's a lot of debate about the best method of steak cooking, so I encourage you to try several to find the one that best suits you.

It's hundreds of thousands of years old grilling meat over a flame, and it still works quite well. Other fuel options include charcoal, wood pellets, and gas.

Different sources of fire impart different flavors to the meat, and this is particularly true for different types of wood. It is not unusual for individuals to decide which source of fuel is their favorite for the flavor they like best.

Eating grilled meat does not cause cancer, and there is evidence to suggest it may not be credible. Therefore, cooking the meat is unlikely to cause any health problems so it has a slight char. If you can show me the study showing that actual humans with a functioning liver only eat meat with a slight char on it develop cancer, I will change my tune on that. If you burn the meat to a crisp, maybe it's a concern, but, of course, burnt meat is no longer edible, and it's a shame that you overcooked it.

After grilling a few dozen steaks, you'll be getting pretty good at sizing up the situation. Instinctively, you should know when to turn the steak, and how long to cook it to get it to your desired doneness. Be prepared to stay near at all times early on, and watch things carefully. The cut size, the form of steak and the fat content will all influence your cooking strategy.

Another common preparation method is the searing of a steak in an oven. This approach can be the fastest way to get the job done, if you like your steaks unusual.

You don't even need to add cooking fat, because the steak itself can use rendered fat. I heat the pan sometimes, preferably cast iron, until it's very hot; then I bring the steak's fat edge into the pan to create a shallow layer of hot cooking fat. I sear the steak after that. Instead, use ghee or butter, or use animal fats such as tallow, lard, or bacon grease. Learn how to reverse sear the steak to raise your game up a notch, which includes cooking the steak gradually at a relatively low temperature until the internal temperature hits the ideal doneness. Then you put the steak in a hot pan to quickly search both sides and attain the perfect finish.

If you tolerate them, adding spices and herbs will give the meat a nice flavor with any of those cooking techniques.

Sous vide is another cool technique that many people swear in order to get the perfect steak. It involves placing the steak in a plastic bag, and holding it for a relatively long time in an appropriately regulated water bath, as long as 48 hours. When you take the steak out of the water, you sear it with a blow torch or in an oven. The product is an exceptionally tender meat cut with a natural flavour. Yeah, my mouth just waters thinking about it!

Some people like broiling as a form of cooking. Nonetheless, in my experience the outcome isn't as good as the previous options.

Several slow cooking techniques can be used for leaner cuts and roasts; these methods can be a perfect way to prepare a large amount of meat to have at hand. Multicookers such as the Instant Pot and other pressure-cooking tools will dramatically reduce cooking times for harder meat cuts while still producing results close to more traditional methods of slow cooking. Another good tool for cooking a roast is the good old-fashioned oven.

The Air Fryer is a relative newcomer to the food gadget world. I've cooked steaks many times with it, and I can tell that this is a very good option for ease and convenience of use.

CONCLUSION

That said, a common mistake among carnivore newbies in the beginning is in fact not eating enough. They aren't used to eating so much meat and thus don't eat enough. Energy levels are declining slightly. As Dr. Shawn Baker is known to say, "Eat meat like it's your work." A change tip: if you're not yet ready for a full carnivorous diet, you might eat meat at a meal first, and try eating enough to satisfy yourself. If I drink coffee or tea on a Carnivore Diet afterwards, should you eat some plants to top it off?

Coffee is an extract of no-carb, zero-calorie plants. It should be seen as a drug and not a meal. Most dietitian carnivores still drink coffee. I drink some coffee, but preferably only on days that I write or fly. I also want it more in cold months, so for me, coffee intake is a little seasonal.

One great help in reducing coffee consumption is drinking bone broth, especially in cold weather conditions. Broth has no caffeine, but it's delicious, very nutritious and soothing.

Regardless of how you end up following your Carnivore Diet, the main lesson I think is that meat is a critical part of human nutrition. Meat is totally appropriate for many and is extremely health-giving. Others can use the diet as a powerful tool for recognizing food intolerances or for battling health challenges. Athletes may find that going carnivore dramatically improves performance, body composition, and recovery. Many may opt for cyclical use. Others may choose to remain "mostly carnivorous," and so thrive.

I can assure you that going carnivore won't allow you to save the world's broccoli from maltreatment, nor will you get a free pass into Heaven. You will be no more morally superior than anyone else and there will be no change in your vibration levels or karmic equilibrium. But I hope you get to have a better nutritional relationship and know a little more about your physiology.

I'd like to thank you for buying and reading this book and I hope you'll share some of this knowledge with those you think will benefit from it. The Carnivore Diet is an emerging subject in the field of health and nutrition and I expect to see a lot more awareness on the topic soon.

THANK YOU SO MUCH ONCE AGAIN!!!